Yoga for Health

Curative Powers of Yogasanas

N.S. Ravishankar
An Educationist & Yoga Expert

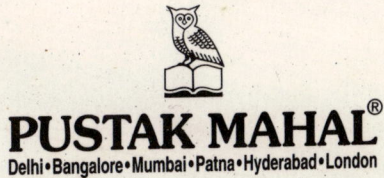

PUSTAK MAHAL®
Delhi • Bangalore • Mumbai • Patna • Hyderabad • London

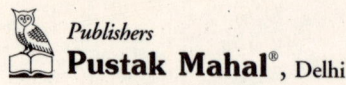

Publishers
Pustak Mahal®, Delhi
J-3/16, Daryaganj, New Delhi-110002
☎ 23276539, 23272783, 23272784 • *Fax*: 011-23260518
E-mail: info@pustakmahal.com • *Website*: www.pustakmahal.com

London Office
51, Severn Crescents, Slough, Berkshire, SL 38 UU, England
E-mail: pustakmahaluk@pustakmahal.com

Sales Centre
10-B, Netaji Subhash Marg, Daryaganj, New Delhi-110002
☎ 23268292, 23268293, 23279900 • *Fax*: 011-23280567
E-mail: rapidexdelhi@indiatimes.com

Branch Offices
Bangalore: ☎ 22234025
E-mail: pmblr@sancharnet.in • pustak@sancharnet.in
Mumbai: ☎ 22010941
E-mail: rapidex@bom5.vsnl.net.in
Patna: ☎ 3294193 • *Telefax*: 0612-2302719
E-mail: rapidexptn@rediffmail.com
Hyderabad: *Telefax*: 040-24737290
E-mail: pustakmahalhyd@yahoo.co.in

© Pustak Mahal, Delhi
ISBN 978-81-223-0724-5

Totally Revised Edition : September 2002
Edition : 2008

The Copyright of this book, as well as all matter contained herein (including illustrations) rests with the Publishers. No person shall copy the name of the book, its title design, matter and illustrations in any form and in any language, totally or partially or in any distorted form. Anybody doing so shall face legal action and will be responsible for damages.

Printed at : Param Offsetters, Okhla, New Delhi-110020

Dedicated to
My Beloved Parents

Contents

Preface	9
Foreword	12
Introduction	13
1. **Classification of Yoga**	17
2. **Common Requirements of Yoga**	21
3. **Surya Namaskara**	25
4. **Yogasana**	31
1. Tadasana	31
2. Ardhakati Chakrasana	32
3. Trikonasana	33
4. Veerabhadrasana	34
5. Utkatasana	35
6. Vrikshasana	36
7. Padahastasana	37
8. Parshva Konasana	38
9. Parshvothanasana	39
10. Garudasana	40
11. Ardha Padmothanasana	40
12. Uttitha Hastha Padangustasana	41
13. Uttanasana	42
14. Natarajasana	43
15. Tripura Harasana	44
16. Trivikramasana	45
17. Ardha Chandrasana	46
18. Ardha Chakrasana	47
19. Vatayanasana	47
20. Padmasana	48
21. Siddhasana	49
22. Vajrasana	50
23. Veerasana	51
24. Suptha Veerasana	52
25. Paryankasana	53

26. Baddha Konasana — 53
27. Mandukasana — 54
28. Sukhasana — 55
29. Simhasana — 56
30. Matsyasana — 57
31. Kukkutasana — 57
32. Parvatasana — 59
33. Mayurasana part I — 59
34. Mayurasana part II — 61
35. Ekapada Shayanadanda Ekahastha Mayurasana — 61
36. Janu Shirshasana — 62
37. Parirutha Janu Shirshasana — 63
38. Paschimothanasana — 64
39. Urdhvamuka Paschimothanasana — 65
40. Marichasana — 66
41. Matsyendrasana — 67
42. Gomukhasana — 69
43. Ushtrasana — 70
44. Laghu Vajrasana — 71
45. Kurmasana — 72
46. Upavista Konasana — 72
47. Navasana — 73
48. Angustasana — 74
49. Kandasana — 74
50. Bakasana — 75
51. Mulabandasana — 75
52. Samakonasana — 76
53. Tittibhasana — 77
54. Urdhwamukha Tittibhasana — 78
55. Viparitha Karni — 78
56. Sarvangasana — 79
57. Halasana — 80
58. Suptha Konasana — 81
59. Setu Banda Sarvangasana — 82
60. Jathara Parivarthanasana — 83
61. Hanumanasana — 84
62. Hanumana Valikilyasana — 84
63. Vibhakta Janushirshasana — 85
64. Ekapada Shirshasana — 86
65. Chakorasana — 86
66. Omkarasana — 87
67. Dwipada Shirshasana — 88

68. Dhandayaman Ekapada Sikandasana	88
69. Yoga Nidhrasana	89
70. Bhujangasana	90
71. Purna Bhujangasana	91
72. Rajakapothasana	91
73. Ekapada Rajakapothasana	92
74. Shalabhasana I	93
75. Shalabhasana II	94
76. Purna Shalabhasana	94
77. Vipareetha Shalabhasana	95
78. Makarasana	95
79. Dhanurasana	96
80. Padangusta Dhanurasana	97
81. Purna Dhanurasana	97
82. Urdhva Dhanurasana	98
83. Akarna Dhanurasana	99
84. Shirshasana	99
85. Chakrasana	100
86. Purna Chakrasana	101
87. Viparitha Chakrasana	102
88. Savithrasana	102
89. Chakrabhandasana	103
90. Ghandaberundasana	103
91. Triangya Mukothanasana	104
92. Pincha Mayurasana	105
93. Adhomuka Vrikshasana	105
94. Vrischikasana I	106
95. Vrischikasana II	106
96. Pavanamukthasana	107
97. Karna Peedasana	108
98. Koundinyasana	108
99. Shirsha Padasana	109
100. Shavasana	110
5. Eye Care—Exercises	112
6. Pranayama	115
7. Meditation	126
8. Index of Yogic Exercises/Herbal Therapy for Various Diseases	133
9. Yogic Exercises for Special Persons	171
Bibliography	179

Preface

With the rapid growth of science and technology, we have seen far reaching scientific innovation, technological advancement, and more than that, the research and development in medical field is outstanding. No doubt the man puts his intelligence for various innovation and research studies. More particularly, in the medical field the scientists and researchers reached the stage to eradicate many dreadful diseases and also developed new medical systems to save the life from various dangerous diseases. Arguing further, our medical experts and researchers claim that due to advanced medical facilities presently available, the life expectancy among the people has been drastically increased. No doubt one can admit that due to scientific advancement in medical field, our scientists and doctors are able to achieve medical remedies for several diseases. But on the other hand, it is not acceptable that only the medical research and its findings have increased the life expectancy among the people. We have read in our olden epics that the longevity, which is based on systematic life practices, food, discipline, control over mind and body, good thoughts, good habits, devotion and concentration which are all the real source to live very long and more than that to live happily during the entire life span. All these concepts that we can see in our Yoga Shastra in order to maintain physical and mental discipline and habits have been explained. Yoga requires mental equilibrium.

We hear the word 'Yoga' from everyone, but unfortunately most of us do not really know what yoga is. Merely performing yogic exercise does not constitute 'Yoga'. It is only one side of yoga, which is related to physical concept. Yogic science has contained several concepts, methods, and regulations, which is very much essential to each and everyone. It should be clearly understood that yoga is a real source to lead a well-knit life. The origin of yoga is very old and has very rich traditional values. We do not know exactly the origin of yoga, but about 300 AD the sage Pathanjali wrote the traditional text on yoga which is popularly known as **'Pathanjali's Yoga Shastra.** This is the first authoritative text on yoga.

The main theme of **Yoga Shastra** is based on achieving Atma Sakshatkara(self-realisation) and attaining control over the mind (Ekagratha). At the outset, one can find it difficult to attain the self-realisation or even control of mind easily. It is with systematic way of life, discipline, and principles one can attain self-realisation and control over his mind. In this materialistic world, very often we are witnessing hatred, violence, unrest, jealousy, discrimination, injustice, torture, humiliation and many other unpleasant events in all parts of the world. People now totally ignore the discipline, truth, and systematic way of life, morality, and honesty. We are witnessing human killings everywhere in the world. No scientific research or medical advancement is able to resist such unpleasant events. Because man has lost his decision making power and more than that, control over his mind and body which provides discipline and systematic pattern of life. But our people have to become aware of the importance of yoga and it should be adopted in their life in order to eradicate all the social evils.

Unlike other books, here an attempt has been made to explain the concept of yoga and its significance in a very simple manner so that it will be very easy to follow the concept. I have made a very honest attempt to educate our readers to know the importance of yoga so that it could be adopted in their life. After several years of experience and research, I have prepared this book with utmost care and attention. I have explained yoga, pranayama and meditation along with illustrations with an explanation of therapeutic advantages of various yogic exercises. This helps readers and practitioners to refer them easily. The constant and regular practice of yoga will help to eliminate all the ill-health and give the real experience of pleasure of life. Sage Pathanjali, the founder of **"Hatha Yoga Darshana"** has narrated the eight-fold path, they are;

1. **Yama** {self-discipline}
2. **Niyama** {the rules}
3. **Asana** {yogic postures}
4. **Pranayama** {regulated breath}
5. **Pratyahara** {sense detachment}
6. **Dharana** {inner abstraction}
7. **Dhyana** {meditation}
8. **Samadhi** {state of bliss}.

All the eight-fold paths envisaged by Maharshi Pathanjali are the universal commandants required for all human beings are included in **Yoga Shastra**. The principles, disciplines, systems and spiritual values, which are very much required for maintaining human values. Thus, Yoga is not only the physical concept, but is more than that, it controls the mind, body and the entire human actions and reactions.

I have incorporated all these information in this book. Though this book contains all these information, I can not say that this work is exhaustive and complete. **Yoga Shastra** is a branch of study, which has several concepts, dealt at length by Sage Pathanjali. Here an attempt has been made to give useful information on Yoga. In this book over 100 yogic exercises have been explained along with illustrations in a simple manner. The importance of pranayama, meditation, suryanamaskar has also been explained. I have given the beautiful photographs of yogic exercises, which help to follow them easily. Those yogic performances belong to Mr. B.O. Sudarshan, (M.B.A.) a renowned yoga practitioner, yoga teacher and more than that he has dedicated his life for yoga. He has received several national and international awards for his outstanding performance and also successfully organised several yoga camps and yoga presentation in and around India. His help and cooperation helped me very much to prepare this book. I am sincerely thankful to him for his valuable support.

I offer this book to my beloved parents whose support, guidance and affection has immensely helped me to come out successful in my life. I am ever grateful to my parents. My respects to my great teacher Mr. Ananthapadmanabhachar, who is instrumental for all my success and efforts. I am indebted to my brother, my wife, son and my colleagues of the bank who encouraged me at each and every step. I am very grateful to all of them. My respects to Mr. Abid Ali, (Managing Director) and staff members of Pace Computers, Bhadravathi who have taken lot of pains to give good computer output. I am very happy that M/s. Pustak Mahal is doing excellent job in the publication field. They have given an opportunity to publish this useful book. My sincere respects to them. Finally I would be very grateful to all the readers, if they adopt yoga and practise them regularly. It is ultimately the reader's opinion about this book that will help me to improve this volume in the next edition.

N.S. Ravishankar

Foreword

Yoga plays a very prominent role in shaping one's life. Practising yoga requires necessary information and guidance. In this book Mr. N.S. Ravishankar has incorporated all the useful information on Yoga, practice of Pranayama along with illustrations. Separate chapters covering 100 yogic exercises, Suryanamaskara and its significance and Pranayama help the readers in finding ready reference. A therapeutic advantage for each yogic exercise will be very useful to the readers. The author N.S. Ravishankar, expert in Yoga, provides all the information in this outstanding book **Yoga for Health.**

K. Raghavendra. R. Pai,
M.A.,D.Y.Ed.

Director,
SDM Yoga and Moral
Education Project,
Sri. Dharmasthala.
KARNATAKA

Introduction

Everyone desires good health and it is the ultimate objective for utmost happiness in the life. Good habits are the essential factors for maintaining good health and each and everyone has to follow good health-practices in their routine life. In fact minor health disorders are quite common to all. In the case of major health problems the precautionary measures are plenty. Some people control their diseases like Blood Pressure, Diabetes, Acidity, Asthma, Rheumatism etc, by taking medicines regularly. But such practice does not in any way completely eliminate the health disorder. On the other hand, it leads to several other adverse health problems. The continuous, systematic and regular practice of yoga is an effective tool to maintain good health and also has an effect to eliminate all the dreadful diseases from the human body.

Though yoga has such a potential power, which adds more health, more vigour, still most people have lack of knowledge of systematic practice of yoga. Most of them perform yogic exercises for a short period, and as and when the health improves they discontinue the yoga practice. For this reason the effective results of yogic practices can not be determined perfectly. Many scientists, doctors, psychologists etc. all over the world are extensively studying the beneficial aspects of yoga which give us encouraging results of positive health through yoga. Before knowing what is yoga, one has to be aware that yogic practices not only give positive health but also help to develop concentration and strengthen the immune system.

What is yoga? The answer is very wide, it is both physical and mental. The term 'yoga' which is derived from the root word, 'yui' means, to join or yoke. This means yoga is a systematic and methodical process to control and develop the mind and body to attain good health, balance of mind and self-realization.

In **Bhagavad-Gita** yoga refers

> 'Natyasnatastu yogosti na chikantam anasnath;
> Nacatisvapnasilasya jagrato naivacarjuna'

That is "yoga is not for one who overeats, neither for one who over fasts, nor for these who sleep too much, and also not for one who over-wakes."

Further in the **Gita** it signifies

> "Yaktaharaviharasya yukatacestasya karmasu,
> yuktasvapnavabodhasyay
> ogobhavati duhkhaha."

Yoga is for him who is moderate in eating and recreation, in actions, systematic in sleeping and working and more than that, it is yoga, which ultimately destroys all misery of human life. Yoga ultimately eliminates all the health hazards and misery of human life.

Most people are of the opinion that yoga refers to performing exercises to keep the body fit and trim. But it is more than that. The systematic yogic practices not only eliminate and control several diseases but also keep the mind perfect, clean and peaceful. That means, the yogic practice gives both physical and mental perfection.

In the present difficult living situations, mental agitation, anxiety and depression are quite common. Everyone wants mental peace and satisfaction in his life. Now-a-days many money making organizations advertise regarding the conducting of classes on yoga, meditation and Pranic Healing etc. and claim that these are the sure methods to provide better health. But these institutions impart training for certain periods with an intention to earn money. The real object is to learn yoga and meditation systematically and to adopt them in lifestyle. Then only one can experience the real benefit of yoga and meditation.

In **Atharva Veda** it is rightly said

> "O man, I yoke thy soul that goes to the next
> World through breath, with two carriers
> the Prana and the Apana,
> Through their control through yoga,
> Seek shelter under God and communion with Him!"

That is, yoga not only provides good health but also provides control of mind, spiritual wisdom and self-realization.

In the **Gita**, the concept of yoga reveals;

> " Tam vidyat duhkhasamyoga-
> viyogam yogasamjnitam;
> sa niscayena yoktavyo
> yogo nirvinnacetasa."

Yoga is a state of disunion from union with sorrow. The yoga has to be performed with utmost devotion, determination and undisturbed by depression. It is evident from the scores of studies conducted by several Universities and research organisations. They arrived at the conclusion that yogic practice helps to cure several diseases and to develop the concentration of mind and eases stress and tension. Unfortunately most of the people are unaware of the practices of yoga, that is why they are not in a position to get the benefits of yogic practices. Before practising the yogic exercises one has to keep his mind calm, determined and cool. This will be the foremost aspect to adopt before practising yoga. In **Bhagavad-Gita** Krishna said to Arjuna,

> "The mind indeed is all you say Arjuna,
> but determination helps; and renunciation curbs it,
> without determination, no man can reach yoga,
> but the self disciplined struggling nobly, can achieve it."

That is, the self-discipline, clean habits, self-control and determination are the important factors to keep in mind before practising yoga. The proper knowledge of yogic system, self-discipline, concentration of mind and more than that punctuality in performing yogic exercise are very important to achieve the benefit of yogic practices.

Classification of Yoga

The main aim of yoga is to unite the individual soul, body and mind in order to attain the utmost peace of mind. In **Yoga Shastra,** yoga has been classified into four categories, They are:
1. Bhakti Yoga
2. Karma Yoga
3. Jnana Yoga
4. Hatha Yoga

Apart from that, in the **Bhagavad-Gita,** several references have been made in respect of other systems of yoga, which includes Kundalini yoga, Dhyana yoga, Raja yoga, Bhakti yoga, and many other systems of yogic practice. In the entire **Bhagavad-Gita** yoga system is described as an effective tool to control body and mind. In the present days of disturbance and mechanical living it is very difficult to renounce bad habits, bad thinking and the disturbed way of life. In the **Bhagavad-Gita** it is rightly said;

" Yogasthah Kuru Karmani Sangam Tyaktva Dhananjaya
Siddhyasiddhyoh Samo Bhutva Samatvam yoga Ucyate."

It is yoga that systematizes the body and mind by renouncing all the materialistic ambitions.

1. Bhakti Yoga: It emphasizes devotion and realization of God or super natural object in order to attain satisfaction, happiness and discipline of life. By controlling the mind, one can attain concentration to achieve mental satisfaction. Though the system appears to be simple, concentration and control of mind is very difficult. It is the mind that controls the functions of entire human body. Attaining control over the mind requires systematic practice. In meditation technique, mind control and devotion to God have been dealt in detail in order to attain peace and happiness.

2. Karma Yoga: 'Karma' in Sanskrit refers to an 'action' that is, a superiority of action to knowledge is the essence of Karma yoga. The Karma yoga enables people to act in a right direction which helps to render good service to the society. That is those who have a determination of mind to do the best in their work and render the best services to the society will get satisfaction, peace and happiness.

In our glorious history we have read the great dedication of our leaders like Mahatma Gandhi, Arvind Ghosh, Sir M. Vishveshvaraya and many other national leaders, sages and saints, and scientists dedicated their life with their knowledge and action. In Karma yoga, devotion to action is a means to the end, not directly, but only as leading to devotion to knowledge.

3. Jnana Yoga: This is a system of yoga of intelligence, yoga of devotion and knowledge. It is the knowledge that helps to know the various things of the world and to attain higher and higher knowledge leading to realization of God. The ignorant man fails to realize the reality, more than that he fails to realize his own identity. It is the knowledge which helps to realize oneself, and also helps to provide realization of mind and body.

4. Hatha Yoga: It is a system for attaining perfection of mind and body through systematic physical exercises. The systematic practice of Hatha yoga ultimately helps to attain Raja yoga. Hatha Yoga provides perfect health and control of mind and body. Hatha yoga consists of three important aspects:

- Control of breath
- Control of mind
- Yogic exercises

Hatha yoga not only refers to physical exercise but also the action of body and mind, the various types of asanas and Pranayama. Sage Pathanjali, the great master of YOGA DARSHANA in his thoughts and teachings prescribed the ways and means to attain yogic perfection. In his basic sutras, Sage Pathanjali gives "Eight-fold path" which helps a seeker to realize self and to attain perfect state of mind. Self discipline [Svadhyaya], Observance [Niyama], Body posture [asanas], restraint of Prana [Pranayama, Prathyahara, and Dharana], Dissociation, Abstraction, Meditation, and Samadhi—the 'eight-fold path' aspects of yoga are very relevant even today.

1. Yama and Niyama: Yama and Niyama are the two faces of the same coin and it is very important for every yoga practitioner. 'Yama' that is self-discipline is the most basic and very important to all human beings. One must establish non-violence, non-stealing and maintain self-discipline to attain perfection. Truthfulness, honesty, and Brahmacharya are necessary to overcome the basic desire. Only then five sacred vows of the yoga, that is 'Yama' or self-discipline can be attained.

The Second aspect "Niyama" [regulations explained by Pathanjali which has five elements] includes;

i) Soucha [Purity]: 'Purity' refers to purification of one's body, mind and heart. The seeker is expected to purify the body, his thoughts and motion.
ii) Santosha [Contentment]: "Santosha" refers to 'contentment'. To attain contentment in all situations, one should practise a high degree of austerity. It is difficult to attain contentment in all situations. Sage Pathanjali emphasizes that contentment must be equal and it should be observed equally in all situations.
iii) Tapas [Austerity] : It is an observance of simple and disciplined life with sincere devotion to attain moral virtue.
iv) Swadhyaya [Self-study]: Self-study refers to attaining knowledge by regular study of soul-elevating literature, sacred text in order to understand and adopt those principles.
v) Eshwara Pranidhana: It also refers to Bhakti or devotion to the Lord to correlate the gap between inner-self and the divine-self.

2. Asana: Asana symbolizes body discipline and also serves as an aid for meditation. Among the several yogasanas explained in Hatha yoga, Padmasana, Siddhasana, Vajrasana are suitable for meditation wherein the seeker remains balanced, relaxed and stable to experience the values of meditation. The systematic practice of yogasana provides both body and mind control in order to attain Sadhana or perfection of life. The methods, practice and benefits of various yogasanas have been explained in the later part of the book.

3. Pranayama: Pranayama (regulation of breathing) is the cessation of the flow of inhalation and exhalation. "Prana" is the life force of existence, the art of breathing is more systematically explained in pranayama. Though the process of breathing is natural and automatic, here in pranayama the requirement of systematic breathing helps to provide body and mind control. The technique of pranayama described in **Hatha Yoga Pradeepika** must be properly studied and should be practiced under the guidance of an experienced teacher.

4. Prathyahara: Prathyahara refers to "Dissociation". Prathyahara refers to restoration of senses to attain purity of mind, by enhancing its respective objectives. In this process one should not react immediately to any stimulation of the senses by various external objects. At the outset, it will be difficult to restore the senses to attain purity of mind, but once prathyahara is practiced one can attain control over the mind.

5. Dharana: Dharana [inner abstraction] refers to fitness of mind through abstraction. Dharana is binding the mind in place, that is, uniting the five senses of perception together in order to control the mind. It is in this stage one can set his mind for meditation and by the regular practice of controlling the mind and senses one can attain self-realization.

6. Dhyana: Dhyana (meditation) is one of the methods to achieve mental purity. The meditation (Dhyana) involves control over sense perception, that is, one has to attain control over body and mind. The purpose of meditation is to attain utmost happiness. By practice of systematic meditation one can attain self-control and Sadhana (achievements) in his life. We know that life is divine, precious and most valuable. But this perception can be translated into reality only through systematic Dhyana (meditation) which gives the real meaning of human life.

7. Samadhi: The most important concept in Pathanjali's yoga is "Samadhi" (illumination) which has 55 Suthras.

"Te Samadhav upasarga vyuttha ne siddhayah."

There are many obstacles towards the way of samadhi and powers when the mind is turned outward. If the mind is in the state of torpor, then it should be disturbed. Samadhi is a process, which leads to the realisation of mind. It is nothing but a stage of isolation having complete unawareness of worldly objects.

In yogasana we have read about Shavasana which provides total relaxation to the body and mind. It resembles the concept of Samadhi. The stage of deep sleep without any thoughts or awareness is something like a state of Nirvikalpa Samadhi. In this stage the complete perfection is attained in all consciousness functions.

All the above eight yogic concepts provide for cleaning the body and mind to attain perfection. The very purpose of the yoga is to give the complete knowledge of values of human life and also give insight of self-awareness, self-discipline and perfect control over body and mind.

Common Requirements of Yoga

1. Basic Knowledge: Before performing any asanas one has to acquire the basic knowledge of performing the asana, otherwise all efforts will be futile. In the ensuing chapters the various yogasanas for various ailments have been explained. The user has to go through the various yogic systems and learn them carefully. There is a wrong conception that yoga should be practised only through some guru or yoga master. No doubt the guidance from yoga teacher or master will be helpful for easy practice of yogic exercise, but one can practise through gaining knowledge from the readily available books, video cassettes and other available materials. In this book, an honest attempt has been made to give information along with postures which helps to easily understand and practise the yogic exercises systematically. Further the classification has been made with the beneficial aspect for each disease so that the practitioner can use and perform such asanas more effectively.

2. Time and Place: When the concept of time factor comes there is a universal notion that yoga should be practiced in the early morning. It is true that in the morning time the weather is pleasant and also the mind is fresh which supplements, to perform yoga practice more pleasantly. But there is no bar to practise yoga in the evening. Those who do not find time in the morning to practise yoga can conveniently practise in the evening. The more important thing is one has to regularly practise yogasana without any break. Those suffering from major health disorders and women during menstrual period, pregnant women after completing 2½-3 months of pregnancy and one after delivery should not perform yoga. In the case of caesarian delivery or any person who has undergone any surgical operation should avoid yoga practice for about 6 months. Once they regain the health after operation, then they can gradually start to practise yoga beginning with simple asanas. In such cases, with the consultation of yoga teacher one can conveniently practise yoga exercise, which is helpful to eliminate those particular health problems easily. Here in this book a chart has given at the end in order to know which yogic exercise is beneficial for a particular health disorder.

Though there is no specific stipulation regarding duration of yoga practice daily practising yogic exercise for one and half hours will be sufficient. As explained earlier, the morning time preferably before sunrise is the ideal time for yogic practice. While performing yoga one should select the place which must be well ventilated with good circulation of air. Such place should be free from dust, fumes or bad odour. The place should be kept clean. Yogic exercise should not be done on a plain floor. A mat or a blanket should be spread on the floor while practising yogasana. Pranayama can also be practiced at the convenient time. But the basic requirement is, one should practise under the guidance of a yoga teacher or one who is proficient in pranayama.

3. Food and Habits: It is an important concept that every yoga practitioner must be aware about the habit of ideal food system in order to attain the benefits of yoga. The consumption of food, the method and quantity of consumption, style of food pattern, and taste differs from person to person. Every yoga practitioner has to keep in mind that a systematic practice of food consumption helps to cure the all health disorders. There have been several discussions at different quarters regarding vegetarianism and non-vegetarianism and their advantages and disadvantages. From the various yogic studies we come to a conclusion that vegetarianism is the best option for both yoga and health. Regarding consumption of food, it depends upon the body structure of an individual. It also depends upon style of consumption of food. Many of them have no systematic style of consumption of food, which often leads to various health disorders. Taking food without necessity or hunger, taking too much fatty food, taking food at irregular intervals is often seen among most of the people. Before practising any yogic exercise it is suggested to adopt good eating habits which includes:

a. Taking one meal a day, with less fat and saturated food.
b. Avoid excess use of salt, chillies and spices.
c. Avoid preserved food articles, packed food, food items containing artificial flavours and colours.
d. Consumption of juices like orange, mango, etc. gives more energy to human body. Taking plenty of raw vegetables and dry fruits helps to provide good nourishment.
e. Giving intervals of at least three to four hours once the food is consumed, provides better digestion.
f. Consumption of enough water, preferably early in the morning and at the time of sleeping. It is suggested to take about half a litre of water early in the morning which should be kept in a copper vessel for about 5 to 6 hours.
g. Totally avoiding alcohol, coffee, and tea in order to get the full benefit of yoga.
h. Taking food 2 hr before going to bed is very important.

i. While practising yoga the stomach should be empty. At least there should be a gap of 4 hr after taking the food. One should not take food immediately after yoga practice, at least half an hour gap is required.

j. Water should be taken at least 15 minutes before and also 15 minutes after performing yogic exercise.

4. Cleanliness: Cleanliness and hygiene are very important factors both in medical and yogic sciences. Here cleanliness not only refers to physical but also to mental. Cleanliness is very important to get the benefits of yogic exercise. The fundamental concept of yoga is to clean the body system both mentally and physically and also free from all diseases, agony and depression. In many of the yogic exercises and also in pranayama, which is explained in the later part of this book, mental concentration and equilibrium can be attained by constant practice of yogic exercise and pranayama.

It has been seen that practising a variety of yogic exercises can check many human diseases. To put together the very purpose of yoga philosophy is to provide mental and physical cleanliness to attain good physical and mental health. Cleanliness includes:

a) Massaging and bathing: In massaging system the most available oils namely coconut, castor or til oil should be massaged over the entire body. Before massaging, the oil should be heated and allowed to cool and then it should be applied over various parts of the body. The massage involves percussion, friction, stroking and vibration over the body for about 30 minutes and while doing massage, it should be in the direction of the flow of blood in order to have a good effect on veinous blood flow. The massage should be done once in a week and it should be done preferably after yogic exercises.

The massage should be done first on the right side of the body starting from right foot and then after completion of the right side it should be done on the left side. The basic purpose of massaging is to provide relaxation, to improve the blood circulation that helps to provide the nourishment to the various parts of the body. Once the oil massaging is completed one has to give a gap of 30 to 60 minutes before taking a bath.

Bathing is a system to clean the external body system from sweat, dust and other secretions from the body. Everybody takes a bath as a routine custom without knowing its significance. Many of them take bath either in hot water or in cold water with application of soaps, which are available in the market. The ideal condition and method for taking bath is by using lukewarm water. While taking bath one should clean each and every organ of the body. One should not take bath immediately after practising yogic exercise. A gap of 30 to 45 minutes after performing yogasana is essential.

b) Clothing: The clothing is also an important concept to keep in mind while performing yogasana. The clothes used for yogic exercises should be comfortable to use and should be very clean. The clothes must be free and flexible so that it should not hinder the practice of yogic exercise. One should not wear tight clothes to cover the entire body as the sweat emits from the body and it must be allowed to evaporate or be absorbed by the clothes.

5. Guidance: Yoga is meant for attaining perfect physical and mental health. In the yogic science, since the beginning lot of studies and research has been conducted to know the benefits of yoga on human life. Yogic exercises give a variety of benefits to human body system. Such being the situation yoga should be practiced systematically in order to get the most benefit out of such practices. This means, for perfect practice of yogic exercise there should be a need for perfect knowledge and guidance on various yogic principles and practices.

Plenty of written books, studies and research findings give first hand information about principle, practice and the benefits of yogic exercises. Even in this book an attempt has been made to explain significant importance of yogasana. The regular and systematic practice of yoga helps attain mastery over yogic practices. To perform pranayama one must take guidance and practise under a yoga practitioner.

6. Relaxation: Relaxation is an important concept of yogic science. Here the relaxation refers to both mental and physical relaxation. Most of them have thought that yoga is to reduce weight or to get some physical exercise. The main aim and purpose of yoga is to attain physical and mental nourishment through relaxation. There are over 100-150 yogic exercises presently available for practice and in all such exercises, relaxation while performing such yogasana is more important than any physical exertion. Even in pranayama, mental concentration and relaxation is attained through controlling the breathing system. The emphasis here is, our practitioner is to get the benefit of relaxation through yoga and pranayama, which is the essence of yoga philosophy. In the later part of this book, particularly in Shavasana the art of sleeping which ultimately provides total relaxation has been explained. The main aim of yoga is to get total relaxation and to ensure health and happiness.

3

Surya Namaskara (Salutation to Sun)

Surya Namaskara is one of the very precious yogic practices which involves both yogasana and pranayama. In the Vedas the sun is considered as a God, to give energy to human being as well as all the creatures of the world.

In the **Rigveda**, 5,29,10 the divine sun imparts knowledge and destroys all evils.

> "The wheel of the sun
> Have two function;
> One imparts knowledge,
> The other destroys all evils."

Further in the **Rigveda** we come to know that the God of universe, that is the Sun provides energy and nourishment to the whole universe. This is explained in the **Rigveda** 7, 45, 3 as follows;

> "May the divine Sun, the lord of wealth,
> endowed with energy
> bestow treasures upon us!
> May he, with his far-spreading lustre
> Provide nourishment to all."

The natural process of sunrise in the morning and sunset in the evening has a lot of impact on human body. They are several arguments that the divine sun gives energy through its rays, which ultimately control the human activities. Many religions in the world consider that the sun is the divine God.

In the **Samaveda** 3,9,7 it is described that the solar rays have power of healing of all the diseases.

> "The solar rays drive away diseases
> Dispel malignant thoughts
> and keep us away from sins."

The divine sun is the source of energy to the universe. In the **Atharvaveda**

17,1,30, it is rightly said that the rising sun, liberates the human beings from the bondage of birth and death.

> "May the rising sun
> liberate us from the bondage
> of birth and death!"

As explained above people worship the divine sun in different ways. But in yogic science it is considered as one of the most powerful systems to offer salutation to Sun. It differs from other traditional yogic exercises because it is the combination of yogasana and pranayama. The perfect and systematic practice of Suryanamaskara not only eliminates diseases and human weakness but also provides energy through its cosmic rays, which helps to give abundant human energy and power.

The established practice to perform Surya namaskara will be in the early morning, that is during the time of sunrise. But few of them will perform Suryanamaskara not only in the early morning but also in the evening, that is during sunset. Whatever may be the practice, every yoga practitioner invariably performs Suryanamaskara as a routine practice and also to salute the divine sun to get energy, health and happiness.

PRAYER TO SURYA DEVA

In the Physical State

O Surya, it is through your rays
That you touch me, awakening and
arousing this body from the deep depths of sleep.
If not for thee, this body is mere inanimate object
Like wood; but for the soul that is present
I would also be jada.

Mental State

O Surya, let me have that freshness
that you bestow everyday with the same vigour,
with the same nature, at the same time,
awakening us and leaving us back to sleep.
And even the moon with its cool embers
Is only your reflected light.
Similarly, let my intellect have the same brilliance
As you have; even if it is borrowed through books
It is only reflecting your light of ultimate understanding.

Spiritual State

O Surya, you are the spiritual pontiff of the entire universe,
the sole pivot around which all revolve,
The cynosure of understanding and capability.
I bow down to thee, for you are the
Fire arounding this innate nature in me
To awaken with zeal, to rise to its zenith,
Beyond time, beyond understanding,
Like you to transcend time
And break away from it.

Courtesy:Tattvaloka Magazine

Suryanamaskara, which involves TWELVE steps, starts from prayer or salutation to the divine Sun. It is an established practice to chant prayer to Lord Sun at the beginning of Suryanamaskara. The Vedic chant on Lord Sun is as follows.

OM HARM MITHRAYA NAMAHA
OM HRIM RAVAYE NAMAHA
OM HRUM SURYAYA NAMAHA
OM HRAIM BHANUVE NAMAHA
OM HROUM KAGAYA NAMAHA
OM HRAH PUSHNE NAMAHA
OM HRAM HIRANYA GARBHAYA NAMAHA
OM HRIM MARICHAYE NAMAHA
OM HRUM ADITHYAYA NAMAHA
OM HRAIM SAVITHRE NAMAHA
OM HROUM ARKAYA NAMAHA
OM HRAH BHASKARAYA NAMAHA
OM SRI SAVITHRA SURYANARA-
YANANAYA NAMAHA

STEP I

Stand up straight and place both the feet together. While performing Suryanamaskara it is preferable to face in the east direction. Fold the hands and place them on the chest as shown in Fig. 0.1. Close the eyes and pray to Lord Suryadeva. This is the first stage to offer prayer to Sun.

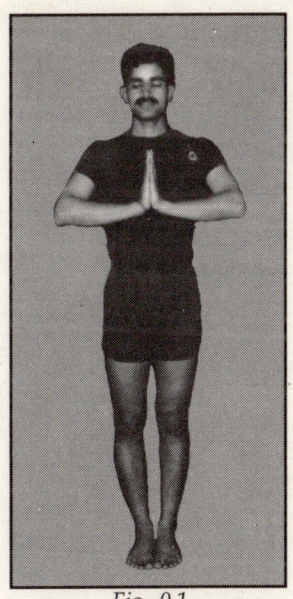

Fig. 0.1

STEP II

Inhale slowly, raise the hands up and then slowly bend backward as much as possible. The legs should be firm and straight (refer Fig. 0.2).

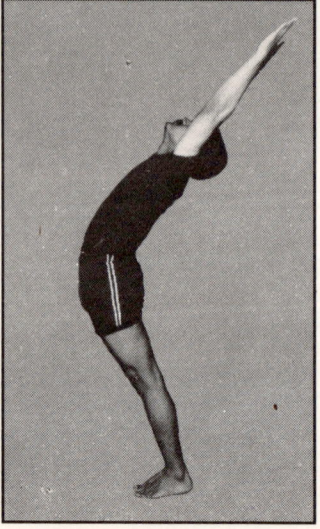

Fig. 0.2

STEP III

Exhale slowly and come forward with hands raised up. Slowly bend forward and place the hands on the ground besides the feet. The legs should be straight and stretched well. Make an attempt to touch the knees by the head (as shown in Fig. 0.3). Initially one may find it difficult to touch the knees by the head, but with constant practice one can easily perform this step without any difficulty.

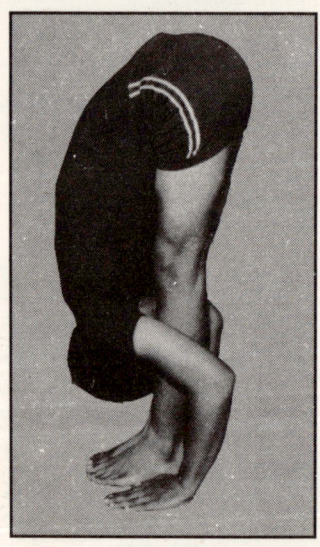

Fig. 0.3

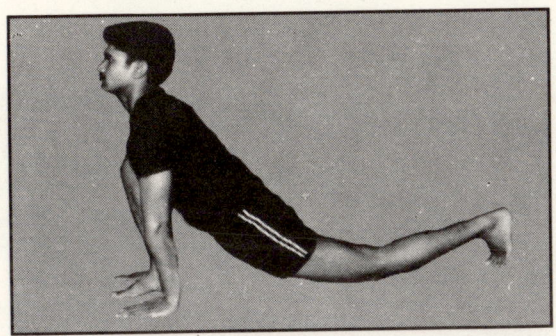

Fig. 0.4

STEP IV
Inhale slowly, pressing the ground with the palms of both the hands stretch the left leg backward to the maximum extent. Hold the head high and look straight ahead. (refer Fig. 0.4)

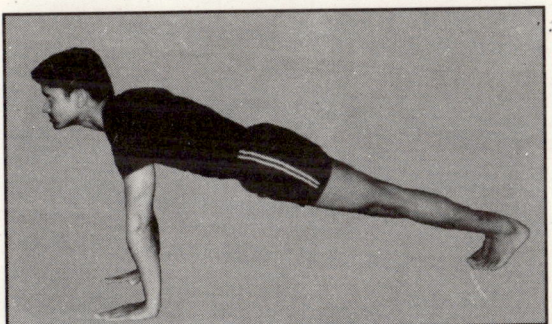

Fig. 0.5

STEP V
Exhale and push the right leg backward so that the legs are stretched well. Hold the head looking forward (as shown in Fig. 0.5).

STEP VI
This step resembles the perfect salutation posture. Here slowly bring the head, chest and knees down so that the entire body should be close to the ground. (refer Fig. 0.6).

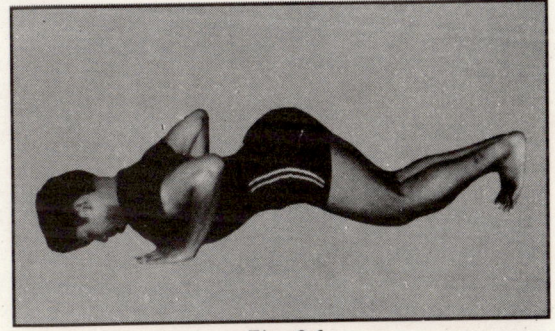

Fig. 0.6

STEP VII
Here in this posture inhale slowly and straighten the hands and simultaneously move the chest and head up. While projecting chest forward raise the head high, bend the back to the maximum extent. (refer Fig. 0.7).

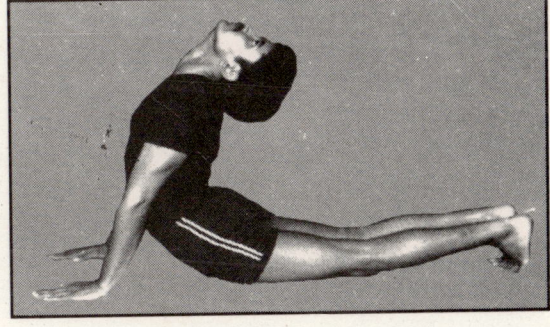

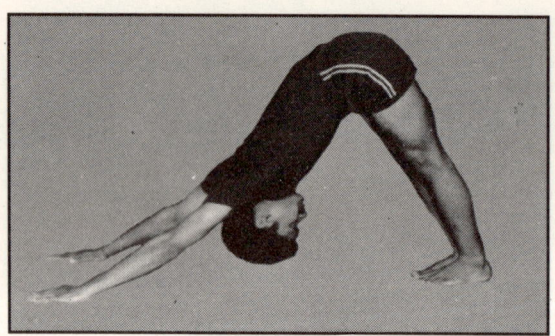

Fig. 0.8

STEP VIII

In this step exhale and bring the chest and head down and slowly raise the waist and hips up (as shown in Fig 0.8). The legs, thighs and back should be straight.

STEP IX

In this step repeat the process of step IV as explained earlier. That is inhale and by pressing the ground with the palms, stretch the left leg backward to the possible extent. Ensure to keep the head held high and look forward.

STEP X

Here in this step, it is nothing but return back to step III process. The head should touch the knees and also keep the legs straight. Perform Rechaka (i.e., exhaling the breath).

STEP XI

This step is a repetition of step II as explained in 0.2. Here once the salutation to Sun has been performed then comeback to the original position. The process will be repeated, in this step one has to come back to the original position as explained in step II, by doing Puraka (i.e., inhaling the breath).

STEP XII

The final step is nothing but Suryanamaskara position as done in Step I, that is, we can come back to the original position, which is the starting position of suryanamaskara.

Therapeutic Advantages

Suryanamaskara is the combination of yogasana and pranayama. It has several advantages.

1. It is a complete exercise for the whole body. Those who regularly practise will get abundant energy and strength to the entire body system.
2. It helps to provide strength to back and also strengthen the thighs and leg muscles.
3. It helps to increase the circulation of blood to the brain and also helps to cure arthritic pain, reduction of weight and tones up the digestive system.
4. Lastly, this is the unique yogic practice, which helps to provide concentration of mind and eliminates mental depression and anxiety. No doubt the God of energy, the Sun will bestow good health, happiness and enlightenment on those who offer prayer to Him.

Yogasana

1. TADASANA

This is the basic and the starting yogic exercise. "Tada" refers to a mountain. This refers to stand like a mountain. This is nothing but to know the correct standing position.

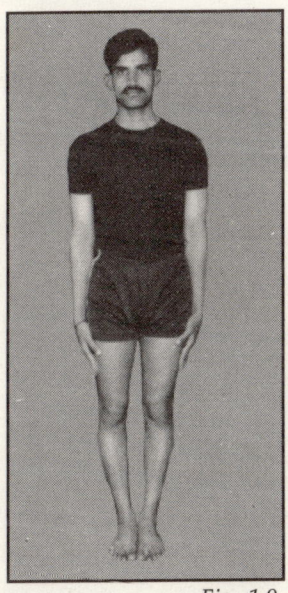

Fig. 1.0

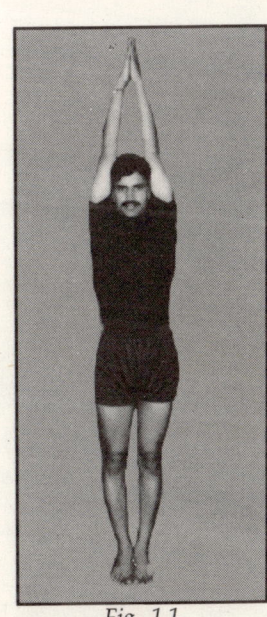

Fig. 1.1

Technique

1. Stand firmly and keep both the feet together. The knees should be straight and keep the hands tight and firm. Concentrate on a particular object and keep the mind calm and relaxed (refer Fig. 1.0).
2. Lift the hands slowly and perform Namaskar (Salute), (as shown in Fig. 1.1). The head and chest should be firm and straight.

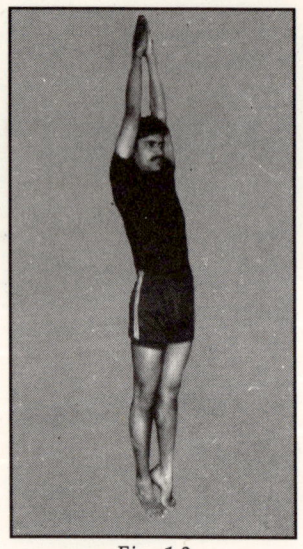

Fig. 1.2

3. Start inhalation deeply, and lift the heels slowly as in the Fig. 1.2. Stay for few seconds and then exhale slowly and keep down the heel to the normal position and relax for few seconds.
4. Practice this exercise for 2 or 3 times depending upon your convenience.

Therapeutic Advantages

1. This yogic exercise helps to give the complete knowledge of perfect standing position.
2. Helps to give control over muscular movement.
3. In this yogic practice the entire body weight lies on the heel or on the edge of the feet. It gives enough strength to legs and feet. It also stimulates the entire nervous system of the body.

2. ARDHAKATI CHAKRASANA

Technique

1. Stand firmly along with legs together (as in Fig 1.0 of Tadasana). Press the heels and feet on the floor.
2. Slowly stretch and raise the right arm above the head and extend with inhalation (refer Fig 2.0).
3. Exhale slowly and move the trunk and right arm towards left side (refer

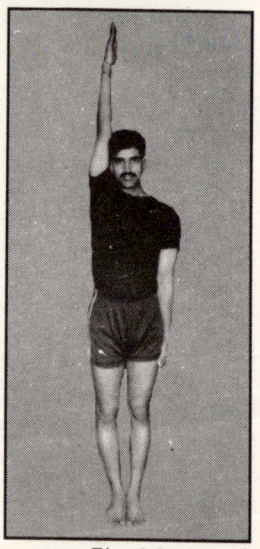

Fig. 2.0

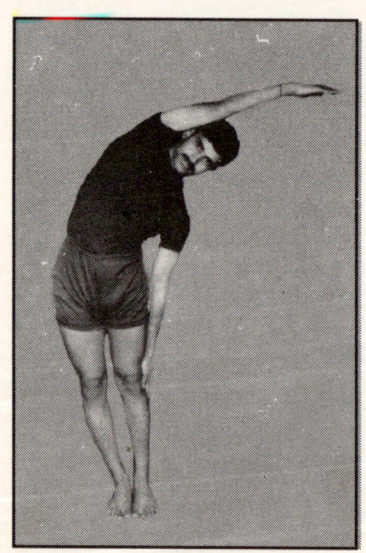

Fig. 2.1

Fig 2.1). The ear will touch the right upper arm. The left hand should be sided on left leg thigh.
4. Stay in this position for 15 to 30 seconds with normal breathing.
5. Inhale, slowly move the trunk and arm in order to come back to the normal position (refer Fig. 1.0).
6. Repeat the same by bending on the other side.
7. Practise this exercise two times on both the sides.

Therapeutic Advantages

1. Performing this exercise will help those who are suffering from back pain, stiff back etc.
2. This helps to promote the function of liver and hence performing this exercise will help to cure liver problems.
3. Simultaneously stretching on both sides will help to eliminate extra fat in the abdomen region and also provides good shape to the body.

3. TRIKONASANA: (Triangle Posture)

"Trikona" refers to 'triangle' and this exercise exhibits revolving triangular posture.

Technique

1. Stand firmly and keep the legs straight (refer Fig 1.0).
2. Inhale, move the legs about 3 to 4 feet from one another. The knees and

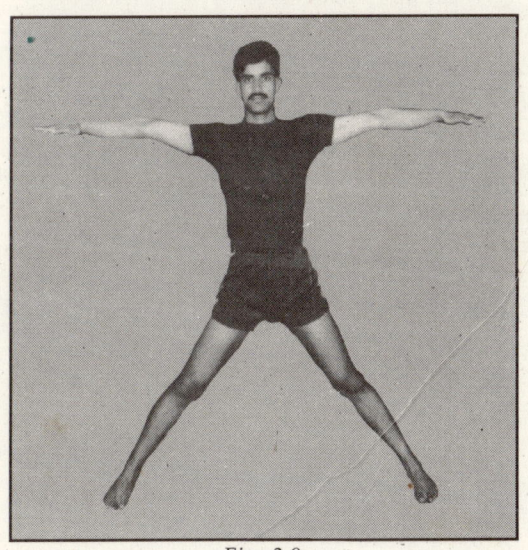
Fig. 3.0

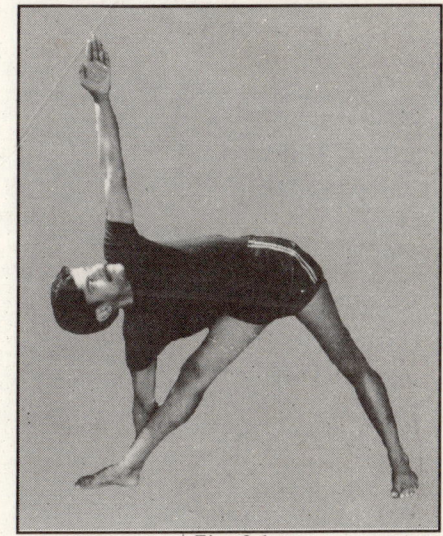
Fig. 3.1

body should be straight. Raise both hands to the level of shoulder to the respective side (refer Fig. 3.0).
3. Turn right foot towards right side at 90 degrees to the right and turn left foot slightly to the right.
4. Exhale slowly and simultaneously lower the right hand palm in order to place the palm on the ground and raise the left hand upward, and see the tips of the left-hand fingers.
5. Hold this position for about a minute and while doing so breathing should be deep and even.
6. After that come back to the normal position. Repeat the same on the other side.

Therapeutic Advantages

1. Helps to strengthen the muscles of the back, hips, and legs. It cures backache, shoulder pain and joints pain.
2. Strengthens the ankles, knees and shoulder.
3. Spinal problems will be cured.

4. VEERABHADRASANA

It is one of the most useful and beneficial yogic exercises. It has a spiritual legend and hence it is called as Veerabhadrasana.

Technique

1. Stand straight as shown in Fig 1.0.

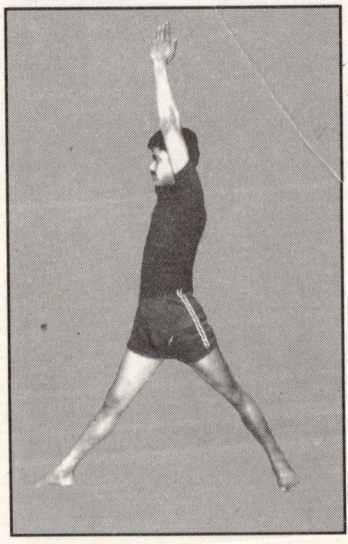

Fig. 4.0

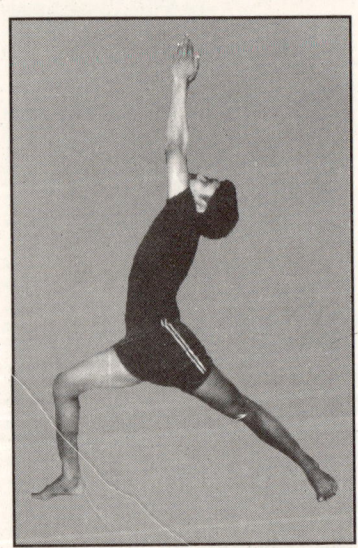

Fig. 4.1

2. Lift both the arms above the head and stretch them firmly. Join both palms together.
3. Start deep inhalation and then spread the legs apart for about 4 to 4½ feet.
4. By exhaling, start turning slowly the body and the leg towards right. Ensure to turn the right foot 90-degrees to the right and left foot slightly to right. (refer Fig. 4.0).
5. Start inhaling, simultaneously bend the right knee to ensure that the thighs are parallel to the ground. Stretch the chest and spine and see the tips of the hand (refer Fig. 4.1).
6. Hold in this position for about 20 to 30 seconds on each side with normal breathing.
7. By exhaling, slowly resume back to the original position.

Precautions

1. Since this asana involves stiff stretches, one should take care while performing this exercise. Further those suffering from weak heart, pregnant women and ladies during menstruation should avoid this exercise.
2. It is advisable to practise this exercise only after acquaintance with other yogic exercises.

Therapeutic Advantages

1. This exercise has several curative effects. It especially helps systematic breathing and ensures good respiratory function.
2. Since this exercise requires stretching the body, it gives enough strength to the shoulder, back, knees, ankles, neck and hands.
3. This exercise is also helpful to those who suffer from obesity and also reduces fat in the region of hips.

5. UTKATASANA: (The Chair Posture)

This refers to sit like a chair. Though this exercise appears to be simple, only by regular practice one can perform this exercise properly.

Technique

1. Stand in position as in Fig. 1.0.
2. Lift the arms above the head and join the palms together (refer Fig. 5.0).
3. Exhaling slowly bend the knees and lower the trunk. While doing so ensure to keep the chest as back as possible (refer Fig. 5.0).
4. Remain in this posture for about 15 to 30 seconds.
5. Inhaling slowly come back to the original position.
6. Practise this exercise one or two times.

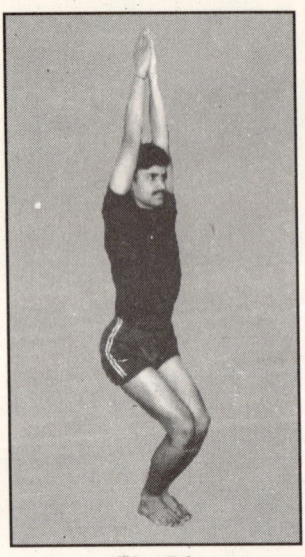

Fig. 5.0

Therapeutic Advantages

1. It is very useful to those who are suffering from stiffness in the shoulder and recurring pain in the knee region.
2. It gives stimulating effect to the chest as the diaphragm is lifted up, which results in good heart functioning.

6. VRIKSHASANA: (The Tree Posture)

This refers to a symbolic representation of Tree.

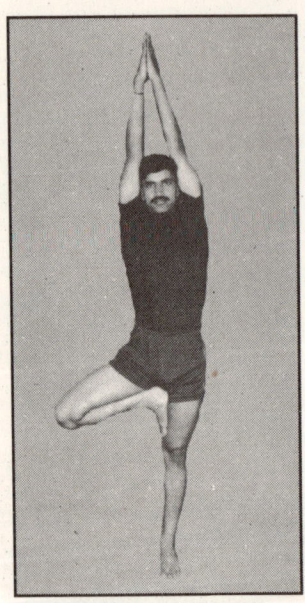

Fig. 6.0

Technique

1. Stand as mentioned in Fig. 1.0.
2. Slowly bend the right leg and join the feet of the right leg to the root of left thigh.
3. Raise both the hands and stretch above the head and join the palms and fingers together.
4. Keep concentrating and focus on a particular object.
5. Stay for about 10 to 15 seconds and breathe deeply.
6. Alternatively practise this exercise on left side also.

Therapeutic Advantages

1. This exercise helps to keep the mental stability and also helps to develop mental concentration.
2. For those who suffer from leg pain, doing this exercise helps to tone up the leg muscles and reduces the knee and joints pain.

7. PADAHASTASANA

'Pada' refers 'foot' and 'hasta' refers 'hand'. Here in this exercise the requirement is to stretch the back and legs down.

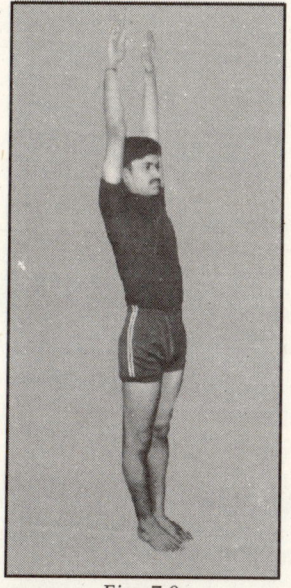

Fig. 7.0

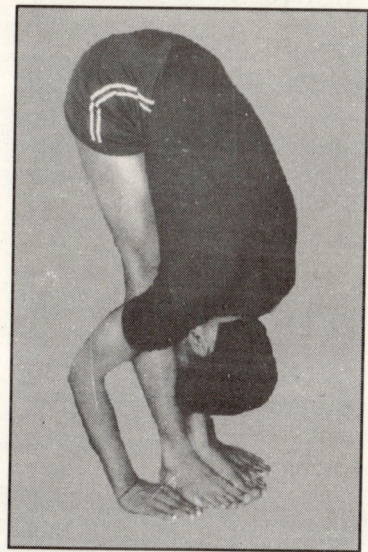

Fig. 7.1

Technique

1. Stand as in position 1.0. Ensure to keep the feet together.
2. Inhale slowly, stretch the hands up (refer Fig. 7.0).
3. Exhale slowly, bend forward and place the palm on the ground adjacent to feet, and now touch the knees with the head. Ensure to keep the legs straight (as shown in Fig. 7.1).
4. Stay in this position for about 15 to 20 seconds and breathe evenly.
5. Slowly place the palms below the foot (as in Fig. 7.2). Remain in this position and take 2 to 4 breaths.
6. Inhale slowly, raise the head and slowly resume to a normal position.

Therapeutic Advantages

1. This exercise gives nourishing effect to the organs like abdomen, liver and kidney.

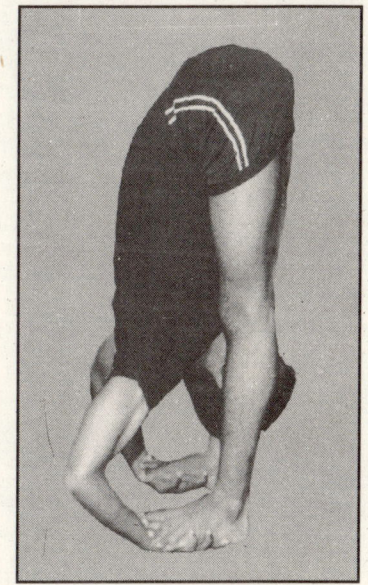

Fig. 7.2

2. Practising this exercise will help to cure all digestive problems and gastric problems.
3. It has a curative effect for back pain and pain in the region of ankles.

8. PARSHVA KONASANA

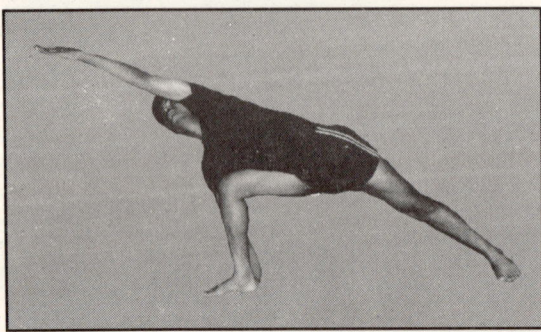

Fig. 8.0 : Front view

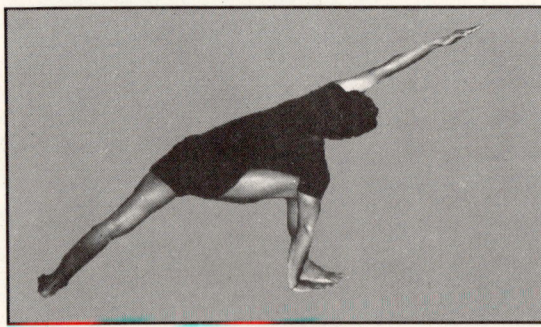

Fig. 8.1 : Back view

Technique

1. Stand as in Fig. 1.0.
2. By inhalation as far as possible spread the legs on both the sides and also raise the arms on both the sides.
3. Exhaling slowly, turn the right foot (as shown in the Fig. 8.0) and left foot slightly to the right so that the right leg should be stretched well as shown in the figure. After that, bend the right leg at the knee so that it should be perpendicular to the ground. (refer Fig. 8.0).
4. Keep the right palm on the floor just on the side of the right foot.
5. Stretch the left arm over the left ear. Ensure to keep head up and focus the eyes towards the finger tips (refer Fig. 8.1).
6. Stay in this position for 30 to 50 seconds and breathe slowly and evenly.
7. By slowly inhaling straighten the right leg and comeback to the original position.
8. Repeat the exercise on the other side too.

Therapeutic Advantages

1. Practising this asana helps to reduce the fat at the waist. This helps to give strength to the thighs.
2. Helps to cure arthritic pains.
3. This helps to cure shoulder pain and chest pain.
4. It helps to provide sharpness to the eyes.
5. This exercise helps to give good body shape and good body structure.

9. PARSHVOTHANASANA

'Parshva' refers to 'side'. In this exercise there will be an intense stretch, more particularly the side of the chest will be stretched more.

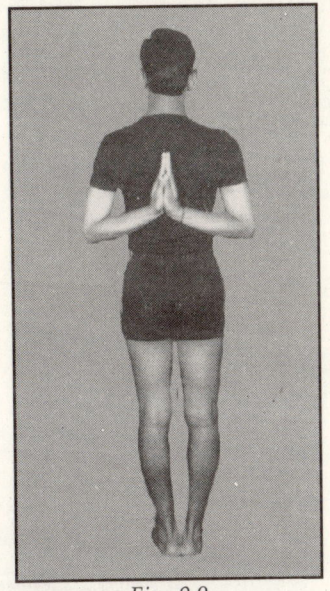
Fig. 9.0

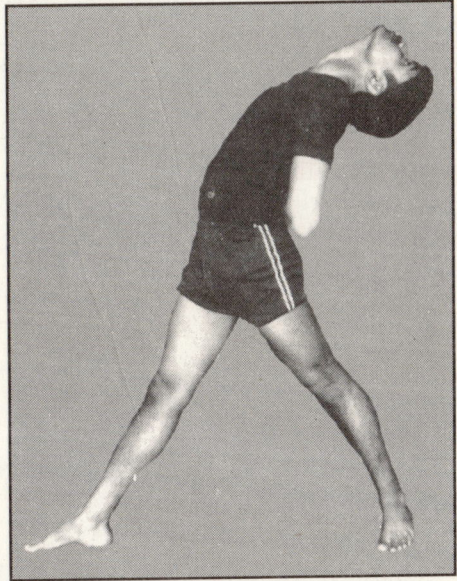
Fig. 9.1

Technique

1. Stand in the posture explained in Fig. 1.0.
2. Hold the hands behind the back (as shown in Fig. 9.0). The hands should be placed in the middle of the back.
3. By inhaling, place the leg forward and slowly stretch the head back. Hold in the position for about 20 seconds. Take about 2 or 3 breaths (refer Fig. 9.1).
4. By exhaling bend the body forward and rest the head on the right knee (refer Fig. 9.2).
5. Stay in this posture for about 30 to 40 seconds with normal breathing.
6. Inhale and move the head forward and then to the original position.
7. Repeat this process on the left side also.

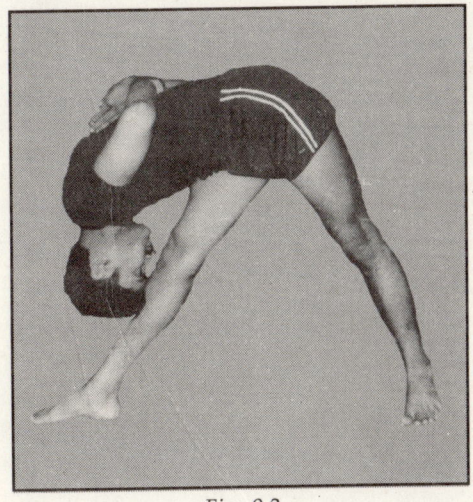
Fig. 9.2

Therapeutic Advantages

1. This exercise helps to cure stiffness of the legs.
2. It helps to cure various spinal problems and back pain.
3. It gives strength to the shoulder and also cures chest pain and pain in the region of neck.

10. GARUDASANA: (Eagle Posture)

'Garuda' refers to an 'eagle'. This posture gives symbolic representation of an eagle. We know that the eagle is the king of birds. Quite similarly, Garudasana is one of the prominent exercises in the yogic science.

Technique

1. Stand in position as Fig. 1.0.
2. Stretch both the hands forward. Hands should be horizontal to the ground. Place right leg forward and take 2 or 3 breaths.
3. Bend the elbow and raise the arm to the level of nose. Simultaneously place the right foot behind the left leg (refer Fig. 10.0).
4. Stay in this position for few seconds with normal breathing.
5. Release the arms and legs slowly and come back to the normal position.
6. Repeat this exercise on the left side as explained above.

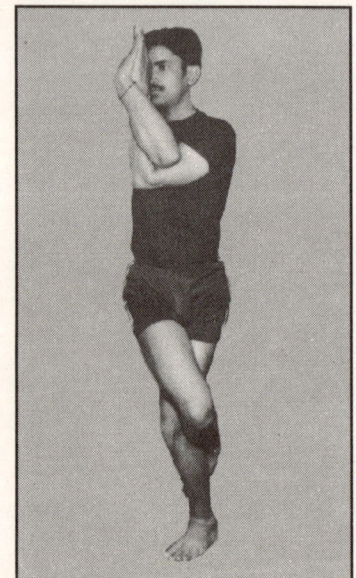

Fig. 10.0

Therapeutic Advantages

1. Performing this exercise helps to provide strength to the hands and legs. It relieves the pain in ankles and shoulders.
2. Helps to remove the cramps in the calf muscles.
3. It gives body balance and sharpness to the body.

11. ARDHA PADMOTHANASANA

'Ardha' refers to 'half', 'Padma' symbolizes 'Lotus'. 'Utthana' means an 'intense stretch'. Here in this exercise, it is half way to padmasana but perform this exercise in standing posture.

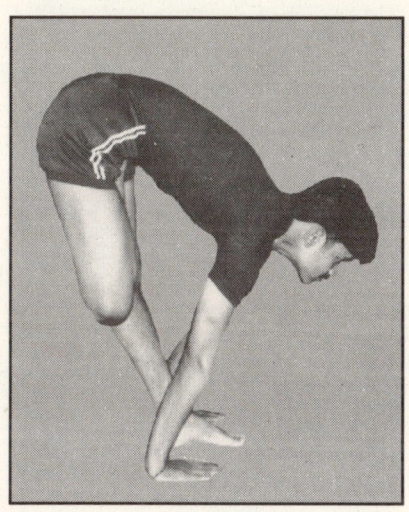 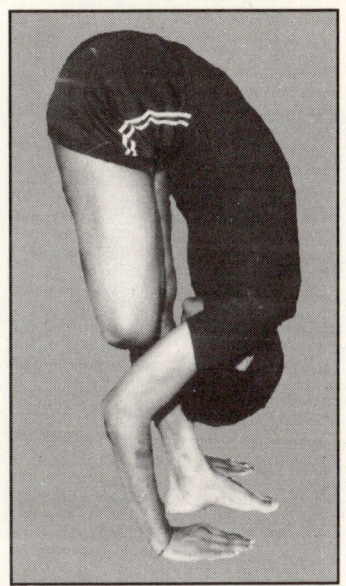

Fig. 11.0   Fig. 11.1

Technique

1. Stand as in Fig. 1.0.
2. Inhale slowly and raise the right leg and rest the sole of the right foot on the left thigh.
3. Exhale slowly, raise the arms up, slowly bend forward placing the palms on the floor (refer Fig. 11.0) and take deep breaths.
4. Ensure to rest the head or the chin on the left knee (refer Fig. 11.1).
5. Inhale slowly by lifting the palm from the floor and also releasing the left foot. Slowly return back to the normal position.

Therapeutic Advantages

1. Helps to cure the stiffness in the knees.
2. Provides good digestive power and checks constipation.
3. Eliminates obesity in the region of stomach.
4. It cures back pain and a stiff back and gives instant relief.

12. UTTITHA HASTHA PADANGUSTASANA

'Uttitha' refers to extend or to project. 'Hastha' refers to the 'hands'. 'Padangusta' refers to the big toe. This exercise refers to standing on one leg and extending the other leg to the front, simultaneously holding the toe of the extended leg.

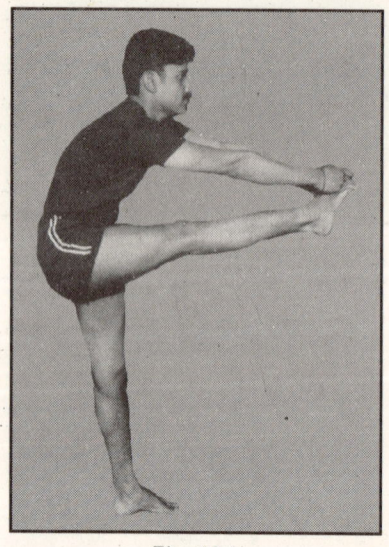
Fig. 12.0

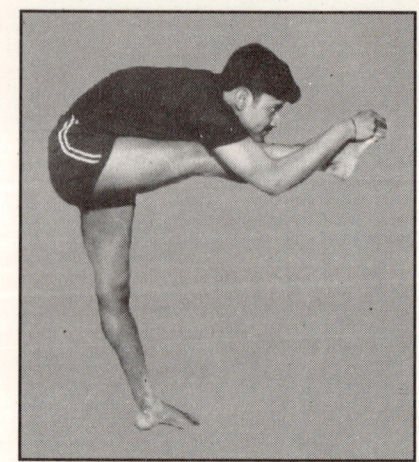
Fig. 12.1

Technique

1. Stand as in Fig. 1.0.
2. Raise right leg up and hold big toe with both hands. Take 2 or 3 breaths.
3. Move the right leg forward so that it should be parallel to the ground (refer Fig. 12.0).
4. By exhalation place the chin on the right knee and take 2 or 3 deep breaths (refer Fig. 12.1). Focus the eyes towards the tip of the big toe.
5. Slowly release the right leg in order to come back to original position.
6. Repeat the process similarly on the other side i.e., left side.

Therapeutic Advantages

1. This exercise is recommended to those who are suffering from obesity and excessive fat in the hip region.
2. This exercise helps to relieve pains in a region of legs, knees and back.
3. This exercise helps to increase the height.
4. Since the legs are stretched in this exercise, it is beneficial to athletes and sportsman.

13. UTTANASANA

In this type of exercise there is an involvement of a good stretch on the back, shoulder and legs, more particularly the spinal part which involves intense stretch.

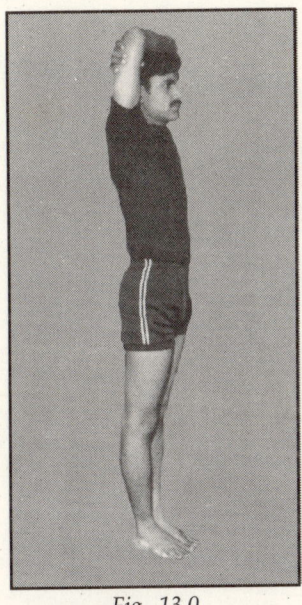
Fig. 13.0

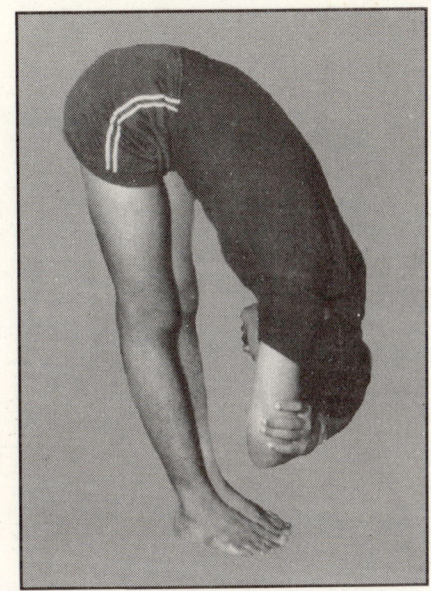
Fig. 13.1

Technique

1. Stand as in Fig. 1.0 and hold the knees very tight.
2. Hold both the hands and slowly keep the hands on the head (refer Fig. 13.0).
3. Exhale slowly, bend forward as much as possible (As shown in Fig. 13.1).
4. Hold in this position and take 5 to 6 deep breaths.
5. Slowly lift the head and the trunk in order to come back to the normal position.

Therapeutic Advantages

1. This exercise helps to give a strong back and also helps to cure spinal problems.
2. Cures stomach and abdomen pain and gives nourishing effect to liver, spleen and kidney.
3. It gives good mental concentration and balance of body.

14. NATARAJASANA

'Nataraja', the name of 'Lord Shiva', that is the lord of dance. This is one of the beautiful postures in yoga practice, which symbolizes the dance of Lord Shiva.

Technique

1. Stand as in Fig 1.0.
2. Stretch the right arms forward and keep them parallel to the ground.
3. Bend the left knee towards back and hold the left big toe from left hand.

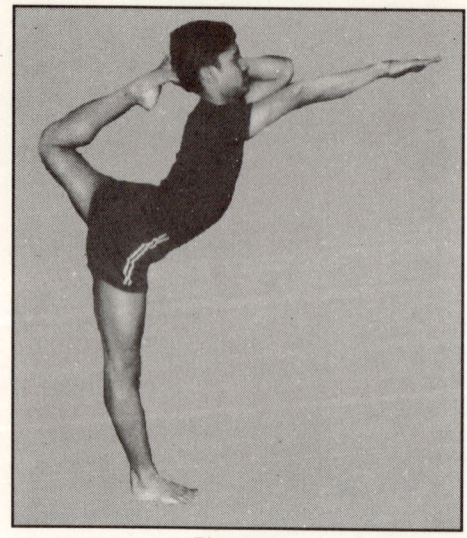

4. Pull the knee-cap up and keep the left leg poker stiff and perpendicular to the floor (refer Fig. 14.0).
5. Keep the balance and stay for 10 to 15 seconds with deep breathing.
6. Slowly release the grip of the left foot and simultaneously lower both arms. Stand again in original position.
7. Repeat the posture on the other side.

Therapeutic Advantages

1. By practising this exercise one can develop vigour and beauty.
2. It helps to strengthen the leg muscles and shoulder.
3. By doing this exercise all the vertebral joints will be stretched and gives good benefit to vertebral joints.
4. It helps to reduce fat in the region of waist, hips and abdomen.
5. Practising this exercise helps to reduce back pain and spinal problems.

Fig. 14.0

15. TRIPURA HARASANA

This asana has spiritual significance and is also one of the most precious exercises in yogic science. It resembles the sacred dance that is explained in our holy scripts. This exercise helps to provide body balance, physical and mental control, concentration and energy to the body system.

Technique

1. Perform Natarajasana (refer Fig. 14.0).
2. Slowly bend the leg to hold the grip from one hand near the ankle region. The other hand should hold near the knees. The legs should be straight and perpen-dicular to the ground. Stretch the body well and maintain the balance for about 8 to 10 seconds with even breathing. (refer Fig. 15.0).
3. Exhale, slowly release the hand first at the ankle grip and then at the knee grip and relax.
4. Repeat the pose on the other side also.

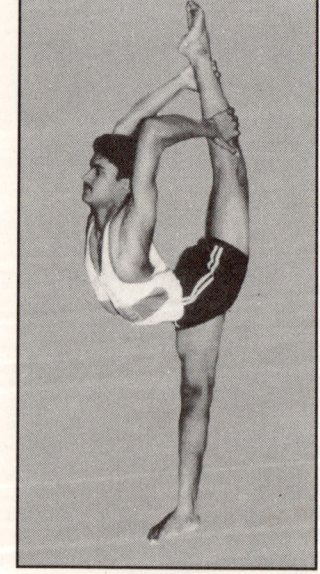

Fig. 15.0

Therapeutic Advantages

1. This asana provides balance to the entire body. There is an utmost stretch to the legs, hands, back and stomach, hence this asana provides stiffness to the body.
2. This asana is most helpful to athletes, sportsmen and also for growing children.
3. Joints pain, back pain, shoulder pain and muscular stiffness will be effectively cured.

16. TRIVIKRAMASANA

This is one of the most difficult and also an important yogic exercise, which has several traditional values. Trivikrama refers to 'Lord Vishnu.'

Technique

1. Stand firmly. Ensure that the entire body should be straight.
2. Slowly raise the right leg upward and then raising the right hand place them on the feet (as shown in the Fig. 16.0). Interlock the fingers and stretch the arms in order to hold the right heel firmly as shown in the figure.
3. Ensure that the right calf is near the right ear and then slowly widen the elbows. While doing so ensure to maintain the body, straight and be well balanced.

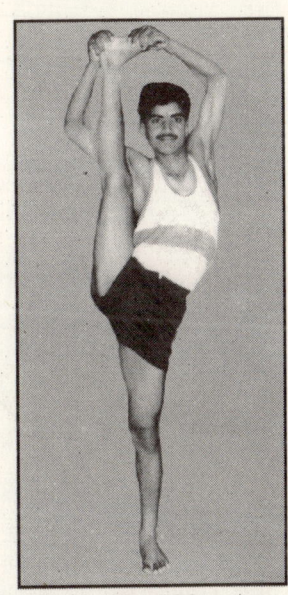

Fig. 16.0

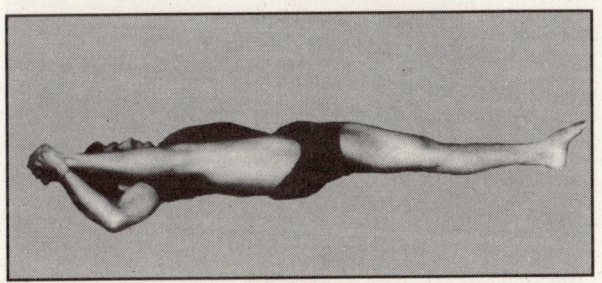

Fig. 16.1

4. Stay in this position for about 8 to 10 seconds with normal breathing.
5. Slowly release the right heel and the leg in order to resume the normal position.
6. Repeat the process alternatively on the other side with the same procedure.

Note: This exercise can also be performed in the lying position as shown fig 16.1. Those who find difficult to perform in the standing position, should start this exercise first on the lying posture.

Therapeutic Advantages

1. This exercise involves extensive stretch to the legs and thighs, hence it helps to provide good nourishment to the legs. This is one of the very useful exercises for athletes and sportsmen.
2. It helps to build legs and thighs very strong.
3. It helps to cure Hernia.
4. Another important benefit from this exercise is that it helps to reduce sexual urge which helps to control the mind.
5. Performing this exercise helps to increase the blood circulation in pelvic region and also in genital organs and keeps those organs healthy.

17. ARDHA CHANDRASANA: (Half-Moon Posture)

'Ardha' refers to 'half'. Chandra is the 'Moon'. This yogic exercise resembles the half moon, hence it is termed as Ardha Chandrasana.

Technique

1. Perform Tadasana (refer Fig. 1.0).
2. Raise the hands above the head. The hands and body should be straight and stretched well.
3. Inhale, slowly bend backward so that the back and hands are horizontal to the ground.
4. Hold in this position for about 15 to 20 seconds. Breathe deeply and evenly.
5. Slowly raise the hands and body forward, then back to the normal position.

Therapeutic Advantages

1. It provides good nourishment to the abdominal organs and digestive system of the body.
2. Practising this exercise helps to cure gastric trouble and indigestion.
3. It provides body balance, stiffness to the leg muscles and to the hands.
4. It provides good body shape and structure.

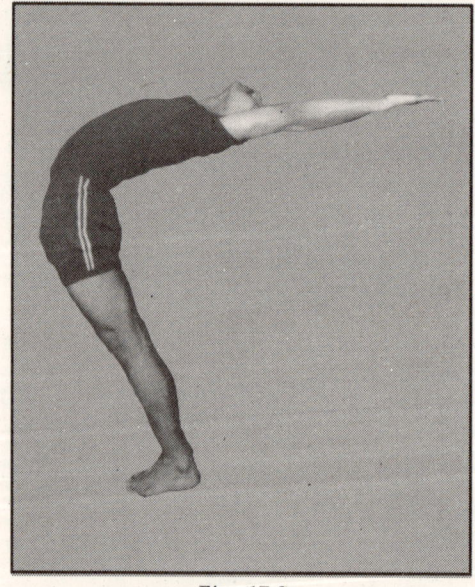

Fig. 17.0

18. ARDHA CHAKRASANA: (Half-Wheel Posture)

Technique

1. Stand firmly. Inhale, slowly bend forward along with hands. The hands should be locked with the fingers (refer Fig. 18.0)
2. As the legs are coming down behind the head, stretch the ribs and abdomen so that arch is formed.
3. Hold in this position for few seconds with normal breathing.
4. Slowly go back to the normal position and relax.

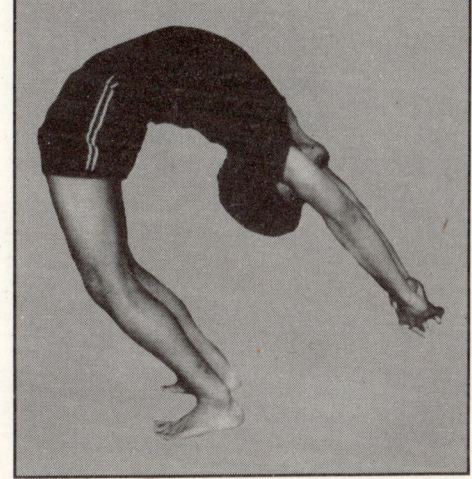

Fig. 18.0

Therapeutic Advantages

1. In this exercise the shoulder, the back, the neck and the thighs are stretched very well. Full body stretching gives good body shape.
2. Back pain and pains in the region of neck will be effectively cured.
3. It provides good vitality and energy to the entire body.
4. Because of formation of arch, the abdominal muscle and chest are fully extended.

19. VATAYANASANA: (Horse Face Posture)

'Vatayana' means a 'horse'. This asana resembles the face of the horse. Hence it is termed as vatayanasana.

Technique

1. Sit on the ground. Place the right foot at the root of left thigh in half padmasana position.
2. Exhale slowly, raise the trunk from the ground and place the top of the right knee on the floor. Keep the left foot near the right knee and keep the left thigh parallel to the ground.
3. Stretch forward and raise the hands slowly. Bend the elbows and raise the arms near the chest (refer Fig. 19.0). Place the back of the upper right arm near the elbows.
4. Hold in this position for about 20 seconds with normal breathing.

5. Slowly, release the arms first, and then sit on the floor and relax.
6. Repeat this process on the other side also.

Note: In the initial stage it will be very difficult to maintain balance as well as twisting the hands. But with regular practice one can attain perfection and balance.

Therapeutic Advantages

1. Leg pain and joints pain will be cured.
2. Due to twist of hands it provides flexibility to hands and fingers. Hence it is recommended for artists and craftsmen.

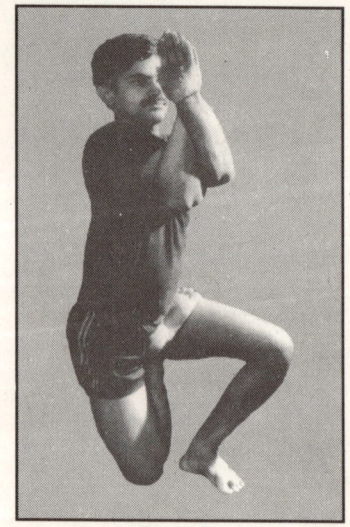
Fig. 19.0

20. PADMASANA: (The Lotus Position)

It is the true meditation posture, which gives utmost mental concentration and equilibrium. Though it appears to be the simple form, the correct practice of Padmasana gives enlightenment to the mind and body. The posture is in the form of "jnana mudra" which represents the source of knowledge. The index represents the individual soul and the thumb represents the universe.

Technique

1. For all the sitting exercises, one has to sit on the clean carpet floor.
2. Be seated and stretch both the legs in front to ensure that the spine is straight and firm. Concentrate on a particular object, keep the hands down on the floor. Breathe in normal position (refer Fig. 20.0).
3. The left foot is to be placed on the right thigh and right foot on the left thigh. Ensure that the heels are pressed against the lower part of the abdomen. In case of difficulty, try to bring them to the nearest part of the abdomen. Stretch both the hands and make a circular shape with

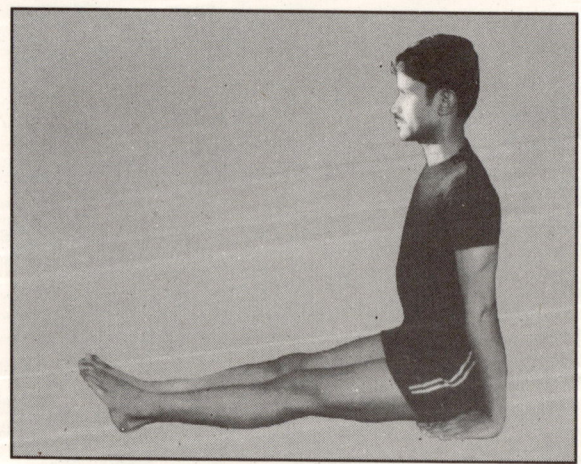
Fig. 20.0

48

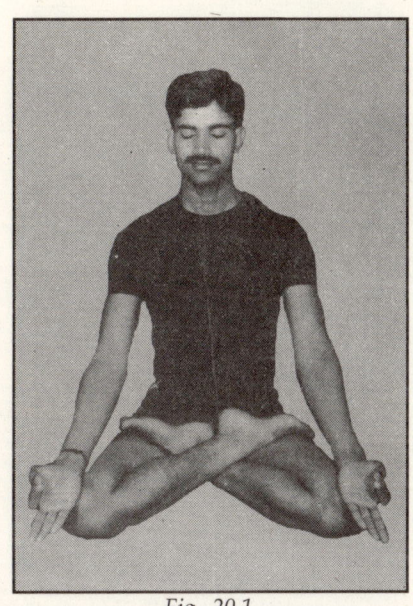
Fig. 20.1

the thumb and index finger. Stretch the remaining fingers and keep them firmly and then place the right wrist on the right knee and left wrist on the left knee.
4. The arms and hands should be tight. The fingers should be pointing to the ground (refer Fig. 20.1).
5. Hold in this posture for about 2 to 3 minutes with uniform breathing. It will be an added advantage to meditate in this posture. Better to close the eyes while meditating.
6. Once meditation is completed, open the eyes slowly and gradually. Loosen the fingers of both the hands. Then slowly lift the right leg with help of hand and place the same on the floor in order to come back to original position (refer Fig. 20.0). After break of few seconds repeat the process by alternating the legs.

Therapeutic Advantages

1. As it is called "Jnana Mudra" the most beneficial use is to give physical and mental stability, concentration and awareness.
2. It helps to cure the stiffness of the knees and joints and also cures rheumatic pain.
3. Helps to reduce fat in the region of thighs.
4. It has good effect on the nervous system of the body.
5. Substantial benefits will be obtained by practising this exercise for those suffering from leg and body pain.

21. SIDDHASANA

'Siddha' refers to 'preparedness', 'awareness' and 'consciousness'. It also means an inspired sage, seer or prophet. This posture exhibits the 'Chin mudra'.

Technique

1. Start with posture 20.0.
2. Fold the left leg back from the knee, and keep near the thigh region. Stretch the toes and ankle of the left leg and bring them in a straight line as far as possible. Place the hands like chin mudra position as shown in Fig. 21.0.
3. Head, body, neck and spine should be straight.

4. Close the eyes and meditate with utmost concentration.
5. Repeat the process by alternating the legs.

Therapeutic Advantages

1. Most of the benefits are quite similar to padmasana.
2. As it is recommended for practice in pranayama and meditation which helps the students to enhance memory power and concentration.

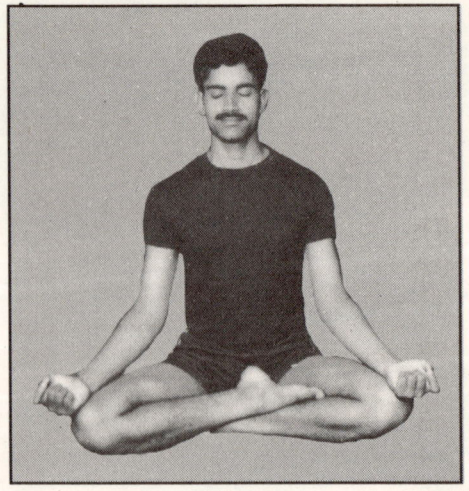

Fig. 21.0

22. VAJRASANA

'Vajra' refers to 'diamond' and this yogic posture resembles diamond. More particularly, this exercise is very useful and invaluable as it retains youthfulness and vigour. The entire body becomes strong like a diamond.

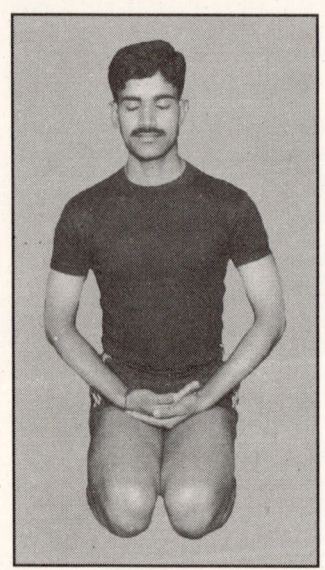

Fig. 22.0 : Front view

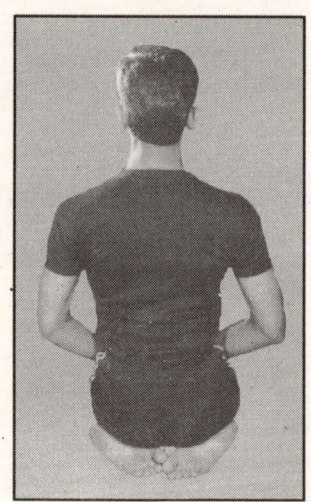

Fig. 22.1 : Back view

Technique

1. Start the position as in Fig 20.0.
2. Fold the knees as shown in posture 22.0. Place the hands in the middle

as in yoga mudra position. Yoga mudra is the highest form of meditation. In fact, Lord Buddha meditated in this posture for spiritual attainment.
3. Ensure that the head, the back, wrist are straight.
4. The entire body weight should rest on the heels (22.0 and 22.1).
5. Close the eyes and start meditation.

Therapeutic Advantages

1. As explained earlier, this exercise provides youthfulness and vigour. The body becomes more and more strong.
2. This exercise is recommended for those who are suffering from weakness of semen and vigour.
3. Practising this exercise helps to cure heart disease.
4. This exercise gives mental equilibrium and develops concentration.

23. VEERASANA

'Veera' means a 'hero', that is, 'warrior', this exercise suggests courage and boldness.

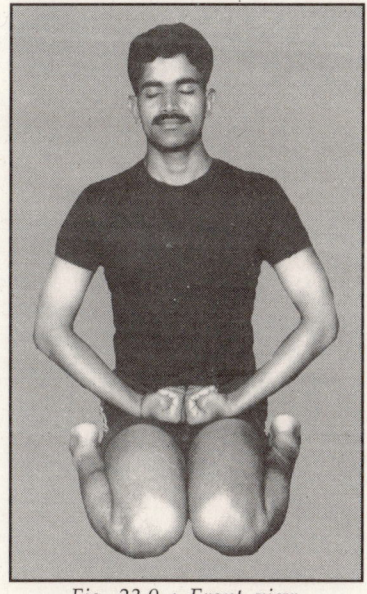
Fig. 23.0 : Front view

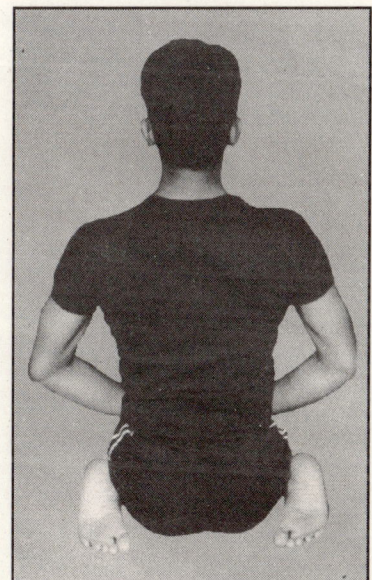
Fig. 23.1 : Back view

Technique

1. Start this exercise as shown in Fig 20.0.
2. Sit as in the position of vajrasana (postures 22.0 and 22.1). Slide the feet so that they are kept by the side of the thighs. The inner side of each calf

should touch the outer side of respective thighs (postures 23.0 and 23.1).
3. Place the hands with clinched hands [Brahma mudra (as shown in 23.0 front view)].
4. Close the eyes and start meditation.
5. Hold in this position for about 2 to 3 minutes with even breathing.
6. Exhale slowly and come back to the original position.

Therapeutic Advantages

1. As rightly suggested it gives enough strength to the ankles, feet and thighs. This exercise is most beneficial to the soldiers and sportsmen.
2. It helps to cure pain in the heels.
3. The Brahma mudra posture strengthens the wrist and fingers.
4. This exercise provides strength to the foot and hands. It is recommended to the persons who are in adventure sports.

24. SUPTHA VEERASANA

It is nothing but Veerasana. Here one has to recline back on the floor, hence it is called Suptha Veerasana. This exercise can be practiced even after taking food.

Technique

1. Sit in Veerasana position (as Fig 23.0).
2. Start slowly, recline the trunk, back and rest the elbows one by one on the floor.
3. Ensure that the back and head touch the ground. Raise the hands forward just above the head (as shown in Fig. 24.0).
4. Breathe evenly and keep the body relaxed.
5. Slowly come back and relax in the original position.

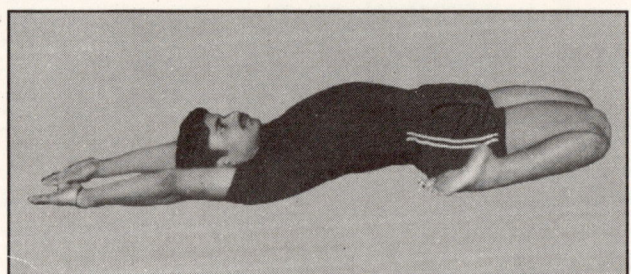

Fig. 24.0

Therapeutic Advantages

1. Practising this exercise gives stretch to the neck and stomach. It helps in good digestion and arrests constipation. Hence it is advisable to perform after meals preferably, at night before going to bed.
2. This exercise helps to give immediate relief to leg pain. Hence it is

recommended to athletes and persons working in standing position for a long period.
3. This is very beneficial to working professionals.

25. PARYANKASANA

'Paryanka' refers to 'bed or cushion'. Though this exercise resembles suptha veerasana, the benefits and the advantages are relatively high.

Technique

1. Start with Suptha Veerasana as explained in Fig. 24.0.
2. Inhale slowly, raise the back, and slowly lift the neck and chest so that there is a perfect arch (as shown in the Fig. 25.0). No part of the trunk should be on the floor.
3. Stretch and fold the arms at the elbows. Place the folded arms on the floor behind the head (referred Fig. 25.0). Hold in this posture for a minute and breathe slowly.
4. Exhale slowly, and then slowly place the trunk and neck on the floor and come back to Veerasana position.

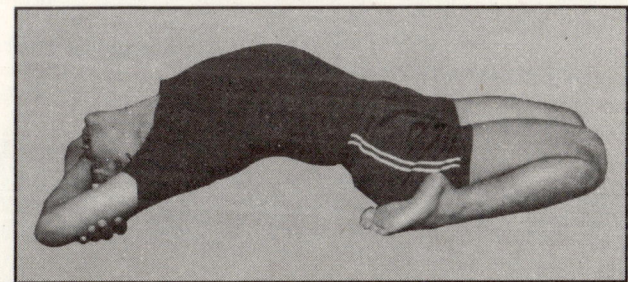

Fig. 25.0

Therapeutic Advantages

1. In this exercise the neck muscles are stretched well, and it also helps to control the functions of thyroids and parathyroid.
2. This exercise helps to expand the chest which will be beneficial to body builders and athletes.
3. This helps to bring relief to those suffering from bleeding piles.

26. BADDHA KONASANA

'Baddha' means 'Bond' or 'grip' and kona refers to 'an angle'. This exercise has several therapeutic advantages, especially recommended for ladies and pregnant women.

Technique

1. Sit and stretch the leg straight (as in Fig 20.0).

2. Slowly bend the knees and place the feet closer to the trunk. Ensure that the sole and heels are together and catch the feet near the toes, take the heels closer to the perineum (refer Fig. 26.0).
3. Widen the thighs and lower the knees till they touch the ground.
4. Interlock the fingers and hold the feet firmly (refer Fig. 26.0).
5. Exhale slowly, bent forward so that nose and chin touch the ground (refer Fig 26.1).
6. Stay in this posture for about a minute with even breathing.
7. Inhale slowly, raise the trunk from the ground and back to the normal posture (refer Fig. 26.0). Release the feet, straighten the legs and relax.

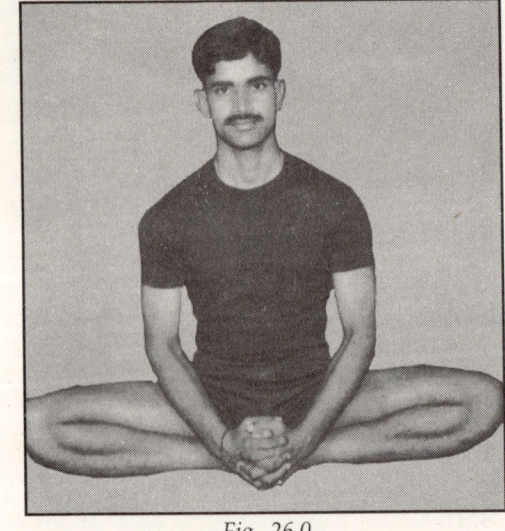

Fig. 26.0

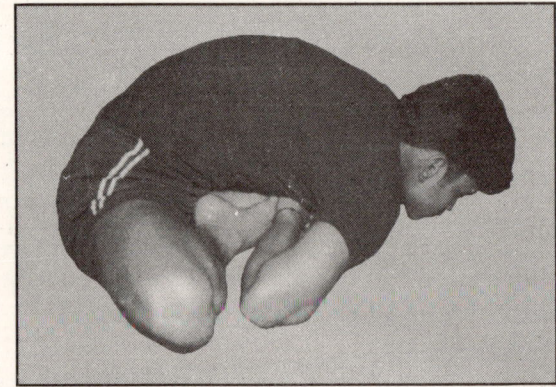

Fig. 26.1

Therapeutic Advantages

1. As explained above this exercise is extremely useful to all women. It controls menstrual disorders and ensures better functioning of the ovaries. If the pregnant woman practices daily once or twice, it will have the beneficial effect of less pain during the delivery and freedom from varicose veins.
2. Practising this exercise helps to cure all urinary disorders. This helps to keep the kidney and urinary bladder healthy.
3. This helps to relieve all the diseases of the urinary tract.

27. MANDUKASANA: (Frog Posture)

In Sanskrit 'manduka' means 'frog'. The action and posture resemble a frog.

Technique

1. Lie on the stomach with the face downward. Start exhaling and raise the legs and hold the ankles with the hands.

2. Take two or three breaths. Lift the head and the trunk above the floor and focus on a particular object (as in Fig. 27.0).
3. Remain in this position for about 20-30 seconds.
4. Exhale slowly and release the palms from the feet and slowly come back to relaxed position.

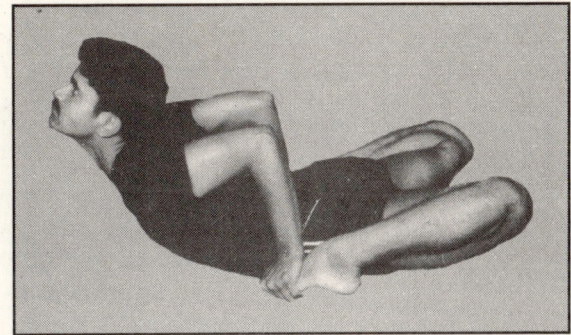

Fig. 27.0

Therapeutic Advantages

1. Since the abdominal organs are pressed, it cures all the abdominal disorders.
2. Knee, joints pain, rheumatic pain will be cured.
3. In this exercise the hands and the feet are stretched, so it gives strength to the hands and legs. It cures sprained ankles and hence it helps sportsmen.

28. SUKHASANA

'Sukha' refers to relief or comfort. Though this exercise appears to be simple it serves as an entry to all the advanced yogic exercises. In this exercise one can start to develop concentration, equilibrium and enlightenment of mind.

Note: Those who find it difficult to perform Padmasana, Vajrasana etc. can start with Sukhasana.

Technique

1. Sit comfortably cross-legged as shown in the posture 28.0. The head and body should be straight and firm.
2. Close the eyes and start meditation.

Therapeutic Advantages

1. It helps to develop concentration.
2. This exercise gives relief from pains in the region of knees, thighs and other joints pain.

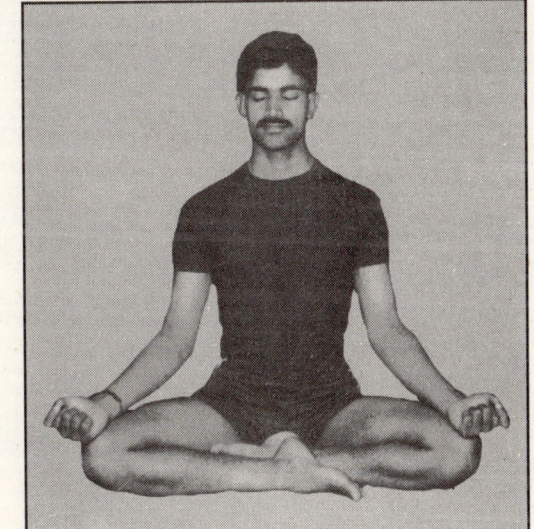

Fig. 28.0

29. SIMHASANA

'Simha' means 'Lion'. This exercise imparts beauty to the face and its regular practice improves the facial expression considerably.

Technique

1. Bend both the legs and fold the knees backward. Sit on the heels comfortably. Ensure the body, the head, and the neck are straight. The entire body weight should be on the toes. Keep the palms near the knees.
2. Exhaling the air, open the mouth slowly.
3. Stretch the tongue out as far as possible.
4. Raise the eyes little, so that the eyes concentrate on the eyebrows.
5. Please note to stretch the hands well.
6. While doing this exercise one should open the mouth as far as possible. Similarly stretch the tongue in order to get good benefits of the exercise (refer Fig. 29.0).
7. Breathe deeply for about 40 to 60 seconds.
8. Slowly withdraw the tongue back and also take back the hands. Finally come back to the relaxed position.

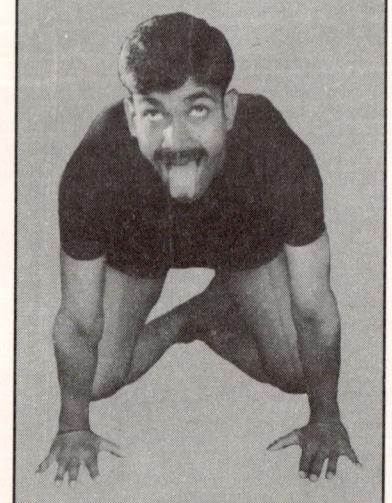

Fig. 29.0

Therapeutic Advantages

1. It is a useful exercise for teachers, singers and musicians as it tones up the vocal chords.
2. Practising this exercise helps to cure throat trouble, tonsillitis and thyroid problems.
3. This exercise beautifies eyes and improves the facial appearance. It is nothing but a beauty aid to ladies.
4. Performing this exercise enhances the sharpness of the ears.
5. This exercise is recommended for those who suffer from stammering.
6. This helps to cure the enlarged tonsils and throat infections.
7. This exercise helps to improve salivary secretions, which in turn, helps the digestion of food. Hence this exercise is recommended for those suffering from constipation.
8. Practising this exercise will tone up the respiratory system of the body.

30. MATSYASANA: (Fish Posture)

'Matsya' refers to a 'Fish', i.e., an incarnation of Vishnu.

Technique

1. Sit as in Padmasana (refer Fig. 20.1)
2. Inhale slowly and lie down on the ground. Fold the legs at the knees and bring the heels near the hips and take two breaths.
3. Inhaling slowly, drag the head back and hold the crossed legs with the hands properly and increase the back arch.
4. Stay in this posture for about 30 to 50 seconds and breathe deeply.
5. Slowly rest the back and the head on the floor and come back to Padmasana position.

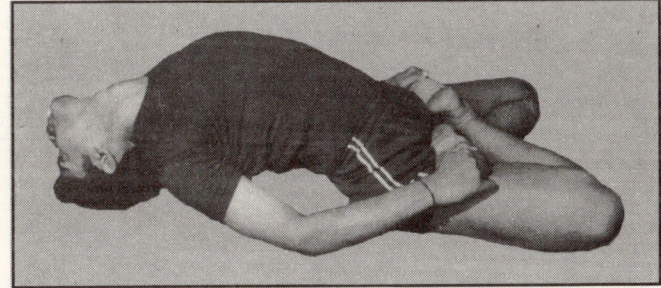

Fig. 30.0

Therapeutic Advantages

1. Since the neck is stretched to full extent in this exercise, it is beneficial to those suffering from neck pain and stiffness.
2. This helps to arrest bleeding in the case of piles.
3. This helps to expand the chest and it corrects the respiratory system. Since the respiratory organs like pharynx, larynx and the lungs are exercised, it is a beneficial exercise for those suffering from Asthma.
4. Performing this exercise will activate spine and back muscles. It is recommended for those suffering from backache and spinal disorder.

31. KUKKUTASANA: (Cock Posture)

Technique

PART-I
1. Sit in Padmasana position (refer fig. 20.1).
2. Drop the hands in between the space of the thighs and calf near the knees. (as in Fig. 31.0).
3. Press the palms on the ground and gradually raise the body above the ground with the balance of the palms (refer Figs. 31.1 & 31.2). The hands should be straight. Lift the head as shown in the figure.
4. Hold and maintain balance for about 20 to 30 seconds with normal breathing.
5. Release the hands slowly and rest on the floor.

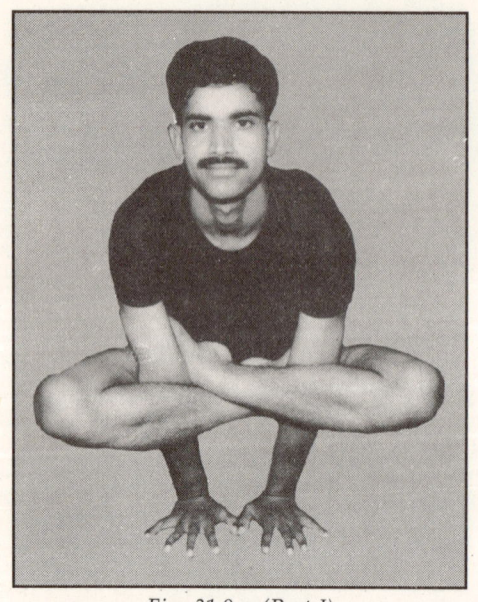
Fig. 31.0 : (Part-I)

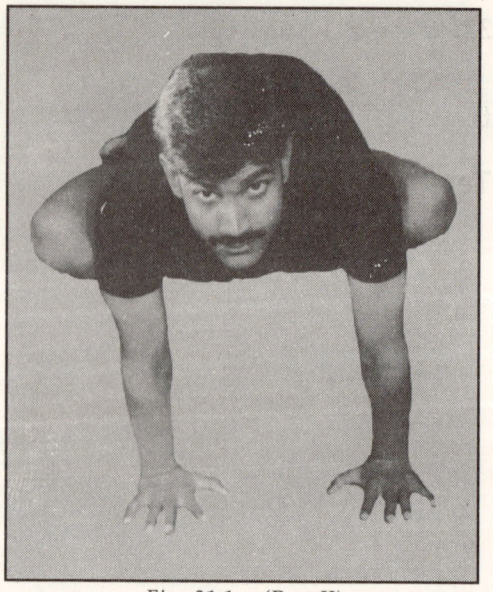
Fig. 31.1 : (Part-II)

PART-II

6. After attaining balance by doing exercise of Part- I, practise the Part-II exercise, which is the advanced form of Kukkutasana. Here in this exercise instead of inserting the hands in between the thighs and calf, they should be placed in front of the legs (refer Figs. 31.1 and 31.2). Raise the knees to the maximum extent.

Therapeutic Advantages

1. Very useful exercise for back pain.
2. This exercise stimulates lower part of belly and all abdominal disorder will be eliminated.
3. It gives enough strength to the shoulder, thighs and to the legs, and hence it is a very effective exercise for athletes and sportsmen.
4. This exercise is recommended for artists and craftsmen because it gives enough strength to wrists.
5. This exercise gives enough strength to the shoulders and wrists. It is beneficial to players.
6. Practising this exercise helps to cure several abdominal problems.

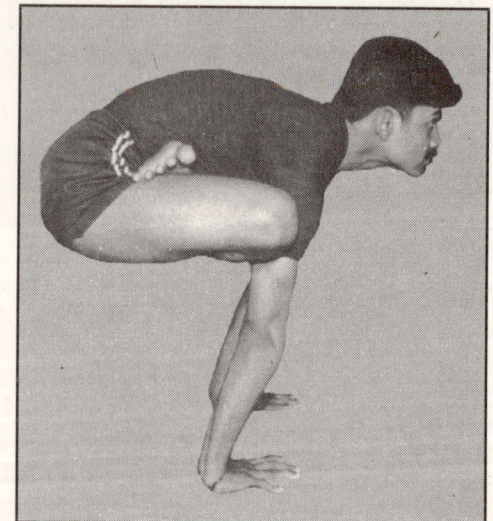
Fig. 31.2 : (Part-II)

32. PARVATASANA: (Mountain Posture)

'Parvata' means 'Mountain'. In this exercise the arms are stretched up over the head and resembles a mountain.

Technique

1. Sit as in Padmasana as in Fig 20.1.
2. From the Padmasana posture slowly lift the hips and thighs so that entire body weight lies on knee (refer Fig. 32.0). Raise the hand up above the head as shown in the Fig. 32.0.
3. Stay in this posture for a few seconds and breathe evenly.
4. Slowly bring the hands down and also rest the body on the ground and come back to a relaxed position.

Note: Those who experience difficulty in performing this exercise can take the support of a wall while doing this exercise.

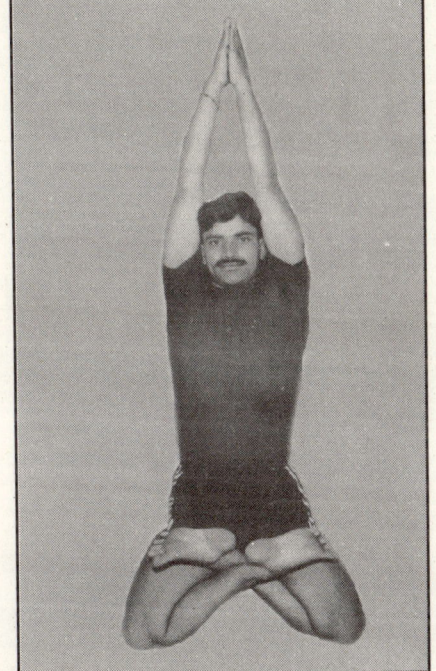

Fig. 32.0

Therapeutic Advantages:

1. It gives strength to the legs, thighs and knees.
2. It improves the body balance position.
3. Removes rheumatic pains and stiffness in the shoulders.

33. MAYURASANA: (Peacock Posture)

PART-I

Technique

1. Kneel on the floor with the knees apart. Place the head and chest slightly forward. Place the palms on the ground so that fingers point towards the feet. Elbows kept firmly pressed against navel point of the abdomen (refer Fig. 33.0).
2. Now stretch the legs backward and lower the head in order to touch the ground and simultaneously raise both legs from the ground. The entire body will be supported on the palms (refer Fig. 33.1).
3. Ensure that the whole body remains stretched and the breathing is normal.

4. Ensure that the head and legs are in one line or the entire body is horizontal to the ground.
5. Practise this exercise for 5 to 10 seconds and once well practiced the time may be increased to 30 seconds.

Precautions

This exercise is difficult to perform and hence it is better to practise this exercise under the guidance of a yoga practitioner.

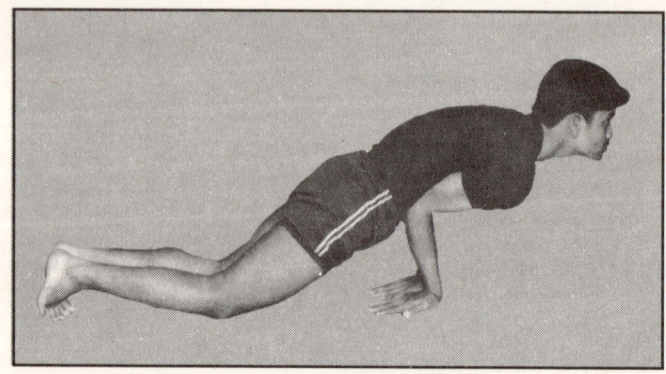

Fig. 33.0

Note: People suffering from high blood pressure, reddish eyes and possessing a weak heart should not practise this exercise. Few people may experience severe body pain or nasal bleeding while performing this exercise, and in such cases it is suggested to stop practising this exercise.

Therapeutic Advantages

1. Practising this exercise gives enough body equilibrium and concentration of mind.
2. This exercise provides increased supply of blood to the digestive system and hence it cures all the digestive disorders. Constipation is cured immediately.

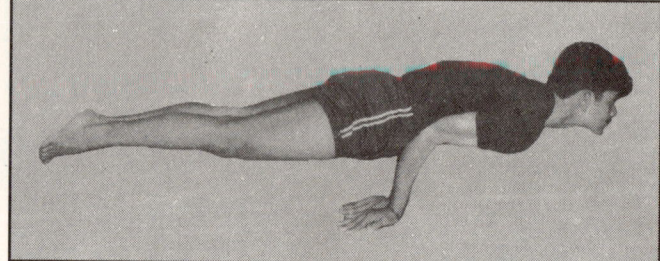

Fig. 33.1

3. Due to the circulation of blood there will be an improvement in eyesight.
4. Performing this exercise helps to make hands and shoulders very strong and hence it is recommended to athletes and sportsmen.
5. Regular practice of this exercise helps to cure impotency.
6. By practising this exercise the problems of liver, pancreas and kidneys are cured. Those who are suffering from diabetes due to the malfunctioning of pancreas will definitely get rid of this problem.
7. Performing this exercise helps to kill all the toxins in the body.
8. This helps to strengthen forearms and wrists and elbows and it cures joint pain.
9. It cures all abdominal disorders.

34. MAYURASANA

PART-II

This exercise is quite similar to Mayurasana. But in this case, Mayurasana is performed with Padmasana posture. Though it is similar to Mayurasana, it gives utmost exercise and stimulation to the abdominal parts.

Technique

1. Start with Padmasana as explained in Fig. 20.1.
2. Continue the process of Mayurasana. The body should be horizontal to ground (refer Fig. 33.1). The whole body balance should be on the fingers.

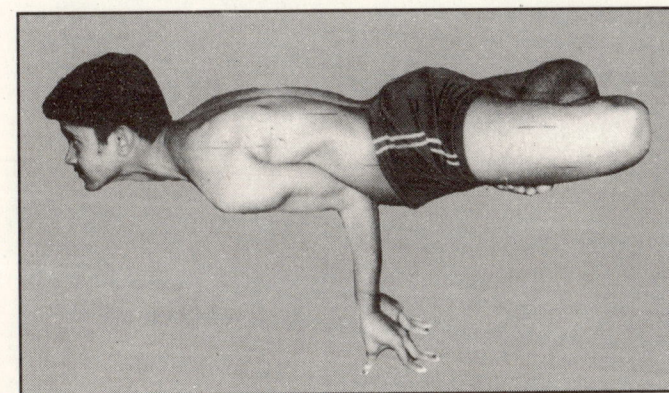

Fig. 34.0

Note: Initially this asana may be difficult to perform, but with practice one can attain body balance and easily perform this exercise. Since it is a difficult exercise, sick persons and pregnant women are advised not to practise this exercise.

Therapeutic Advantages

1. Performing this exercise tones up the abdominal portion, hence this exercise cures all the abdominal diseases most effectively.
2. This exercise helps to increase digestive power and cures constipation and stomach pain.
3. This exercise has curative effect for those suffering from diabetes.
4. This exercise gives strength to the forearms, fingers, thighs and legs and hence it is more effective for athletes and sportsmen.

35. EKAPADA SHAYANADANDA EKAHASTHA MAYURASANA
   (Single Hand Balance Posture)

Technique

1. Perform Vajrasana (refer Fig. 22.0)
2. Stand on the knees, slowly lock the left leg with the support of big toe near the waist.
3. Exhale, put the body weight on the wrist of the left hand. Raise the legs

from the ground, stretch the trunk and head forward. The right hand should be straight and horizontal to the ground (refer Fig. 35.0).

4. Hold in this position for about 10 to 20 seconds with even breathing.

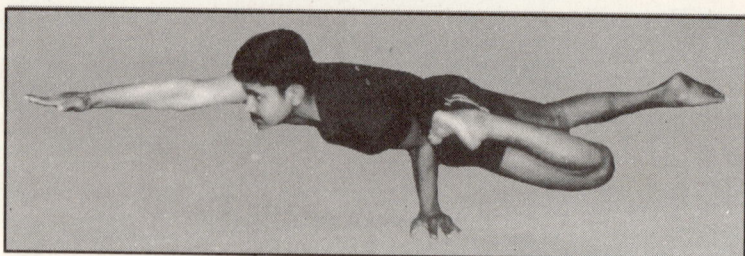

Fig. 35.0

Therapeutic Advantages

1. Though many of the therapeutic advantages are similar to Mayurasana in this exercise as the entire body balance rests on wrists, it gives enough strength to wrists and hands.
2. Abdominal disorders and digestive disorders are effectively cured.
3. Provides strength to the elbows, forearms and wrists. Hence it is recommended for artists, athletes and sportsmen.

36. JANU SHIRSHASANA: (Touching the Head on the Knee)

In this yogic posture one leg has to be stretched out and the other should be at the knee. 'Janu' refers to the 'knee'. 'Shirsha' refers to the 'head'.

Technique

1. Sit on the ground with the legs stretched (as in Fig 20.0).
2. Slowly bend the left leg and place near the thigh of the right leg. Stretch the arms forward and place near the right foot and hold with the hands. Exhale slowly and move the trunk forward (refer Fig. 36.0).
3. Exhale slowly and gradually move the trunk forward so that the chin is placed on the right leg (refer Fig. 36.1).
4. Inhale slowly, raise the head and trunk. Release the hand's grip and straighten the legs in order to comeback to normal position.
5. Practise this exercise for both the legs.

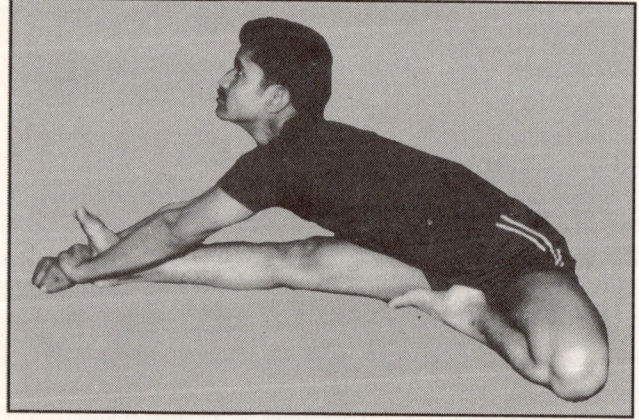

Fig. 36.0

Therapeutic Advantages:

1. Practising this exercise stimulates the liver and the spleen so that it particularly helps those suffering from constipation and indigestion.
2. This helps to nourish the kidneys.
3. This is most beneficial for those suffering from enlargement of prostrate glands.
4. This provides strength to the shoulder, leg and knees and cures the joints pain instantly.
5. For those who are suffering from obesity in the region of stomach and hips, this exercise is more beneficial.

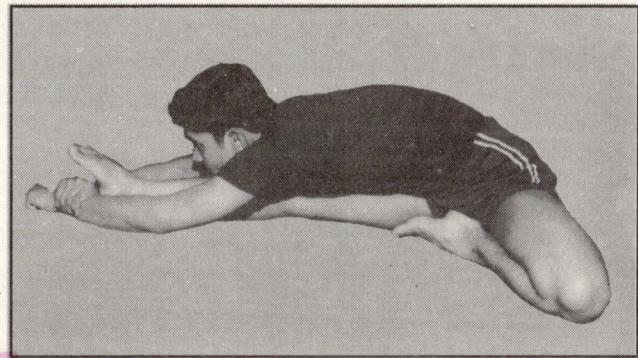

Fig. 36.1

37. PARIRUTHA JANU SHIRSHASANA

This exercise appears to be similar to Janu Shirshasana. The only variation is leaning the body on one side.

Technique

1. Sit as in position 36.1.
2. Stretch the trunk back so that the body is leaned on the side. Try to move the head in order to face the top (Refer Fig. 37.0).
3. Hold in the posture for about 20 seconds with normal breathing.
4. Inhale slowly and release the hands and move the trunk back to the original position.
5. Repeat this posture on the other side too.

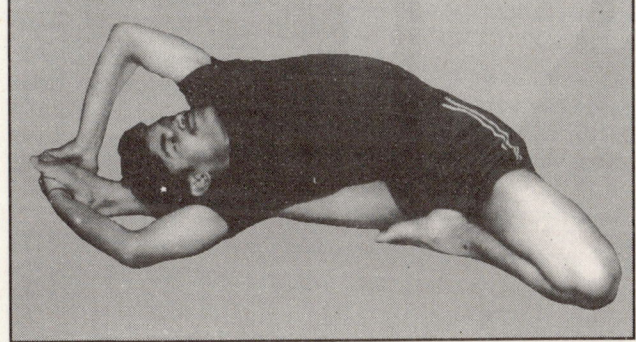

Fig. 37.0

Therapeutic Advantages

1. This helps to cure all spinal problems and the spine becomes more elastic.

2. Helps to cure constipation and indigestion.
3. Practising this exercise cures joint and rheumatic pains.
4. This is helpful to diabetic patients and those suffering from kidney trouble.
5. This exercise rejuvenates and develops the back and its nerves. It is helpful to those who are suffering from back pain.
6. The problems of gall bladder and abdominal disorders are cured.

38. PASCHIMOTHANASANA

'Paschima' refers to 'West'. In this exercise the spinal chord gets more exercise and becomes more elastic. 'Paschima' here refers to the 'Dorsal or backside'. 'Thana' means stretch. The name itself suggests that the back is stretched very well.

Technique

1. Sit on the ground with extended leg forward (as fig in 20.0). The legs and thighs should remain straight. Slowly bend forward and hold the big toes with hands. (refer Fig. 38.0).
2. Exhale slowly and bend the head and trunk downwards till it touches the knee. Hold in this position about 20 seconds with normal breathing.
3. Ensure to hold the toes while exercise is in process. The legs should remain straight and touched to the ground (refer Fig. 38.1).
4. Inhale slowly and raise the head from the knees and come back to the original position.

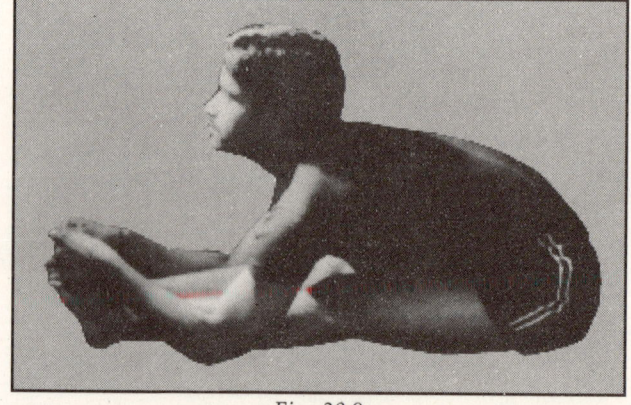

Fig. 38.0

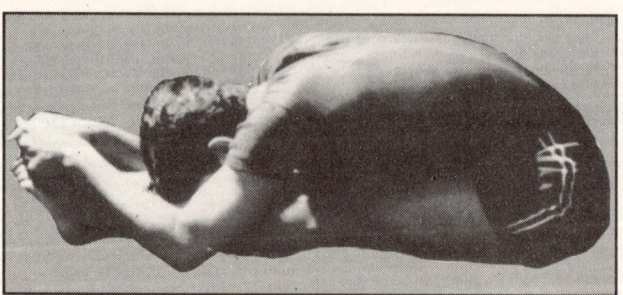

Fig. 38.1

Therapeutic Advantages

1. Since the stomach is exercised heavily, it removes obesity. For obese people though it

appears to be difficult to perform in the initial stage, but with gradual practice one can easily perform this exercise.

2. This exercise tones up the spine, nerve system and abdominal area. As such problems in the area of spine, nervous system and abdomen are cured.
3. This exercise activates stomach, liver, kidneys and pancreas. The diabetic people invariably perform this exercise in order to get good benefit.
4. Practising this exercise helps to better blood circulation and problems in prostate gland, uterus and urinary bladder will be cured.
5. This is an effective exercise for those who are suffering from kidney problems.
6. This exercise helps to cure skin disease and cures pains in the region of the spine and back.
7. This exercise is particularly helpful to those who are short tempered and agitated, mentally depressed and those who are suffering from high blood pressure.
8. Performing this exercise helps to increase vitality and cures impotency.
9. This exercise effectively cures constipation and indigestion.

39. URDHVAMUKA PASCHIMOTHANASANA

'Urdhva' means 'upward'. 'Mukha' refers to 'face'. That is, the face upward. Here the back and legs are stretched well.

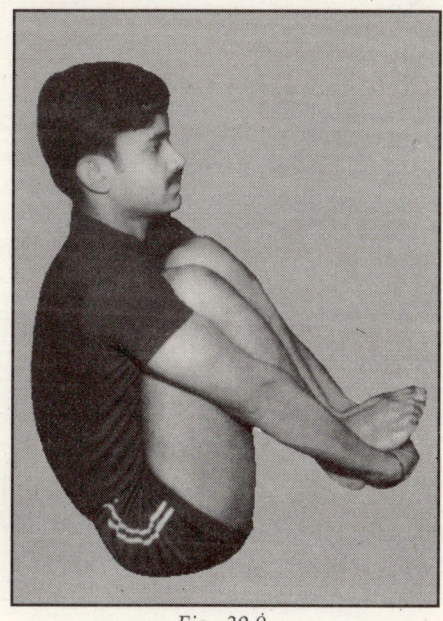

Fig. 39.0

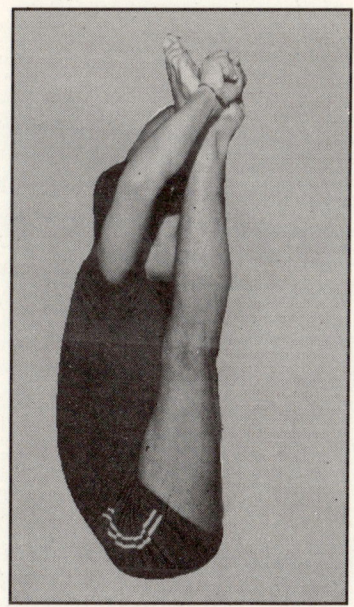

Fig. 39.1

Technique

1. Sit on the ground stretching the legs forward. Slowly bend the legs at the knees and hold the feet with the hands.(refer Fig. 39.0).
2. Exhale slowly and stretch the legs upward. Place the head above the knees and stay for a few seconds in this position with normal breathing. (refer Fig. 39.1).
3. Slowly turn the hands in order to hold the grip on the heels.(refer Fig. 39.2).
4. Inhale slowly, release the hands and bend the leg in order to resume normal position.

Therapeutic Advantages

1. Though this exercise is having similar advantages as those of Paschimothasana, it provides equilibrium and mental stability and promotes mental concentration.
2. In this exercise the legs and thighs are fully stretched. Hence, this exercise is helpful to athletes and sports people.
3. This gives good relief to back pain.
4. This exercise helps to cure hernia.

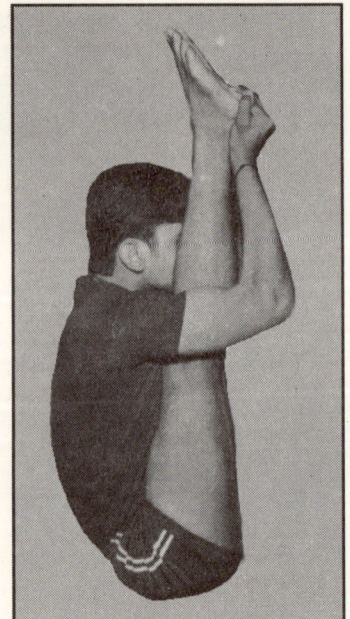

Fig. 39.2

40. MARICHASANA: (Spinal Twist)

Technique

1. Sit on the floor and stretch the legs forward.
2. Bend the left knee and heel should touch the back of the thigh. It should be perpendicular to the ground. Move the shoulder and stretch the arms back and hold the hands.
3. Turn slowly to the left and take a few breaths (as shown Fig. 40.0).
4. Exhale slowly and bend forward so that the chin is

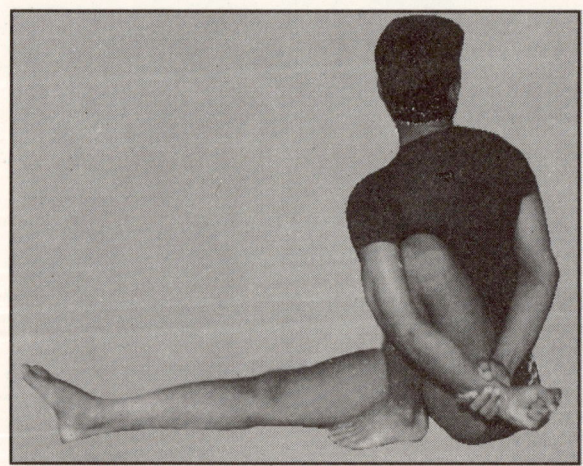

Fig. 40.0

placed on the thigh just above the right knee. The shoulder should be straight. Stay in this position for a few seconds and breathe normally. (refer Fig. 40.1).

5. Inhale slowly, raise the head and relax. Practise this exercise on the other side too.

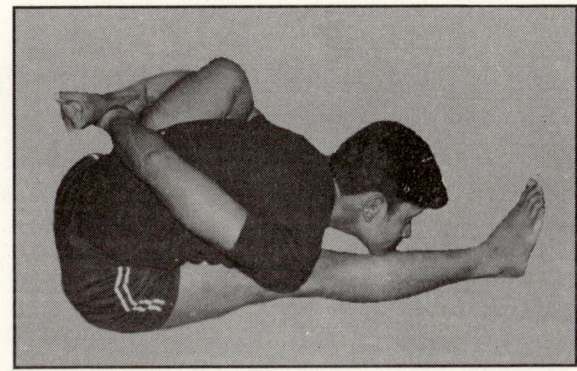

Fig. 40.1

Therapeutic Advantages

1. Practising this exercise helps to cure all the spinal problems.
2. This is a useful exercise for those who are suffering from gall-bladder and kidney problems.
3. It is a good exercise for diabetic patients.
4. This helps to cure shoulder pain and slipped disc.
5. Helps to maintain good blood circulation in the abdominal region and keeps them healthy.

41. MATSYENDRASANA: (Yogi Matsyendra Posture)

A. Ardha Matsyendrasana : We know that Matsyendra is the founder of Hatha Vidhya whose contribution to the yogic science is rich and varied. 'Ardha' means 'half' and 'Matsyendra' refers to 'Lord of fishes'.

Technique

1. Sit on the left leg which is to be bended towards back so as to place under the hips between the anus and genital organ.
2. Place the right leg towards side of the left leg and place both on the ground. (refer Fig. 41.0).
3. Slowly turn the head back by stretching the right arm (refer Fig. 41.1)
4. Ensure to turn the trunk about 90 degrees to the left, placing the right hand arm on the thighs of left leg (refer Fig. 41.2)
5. Remain in this pose for a few seconds and alternatively practise the posture on the other side.

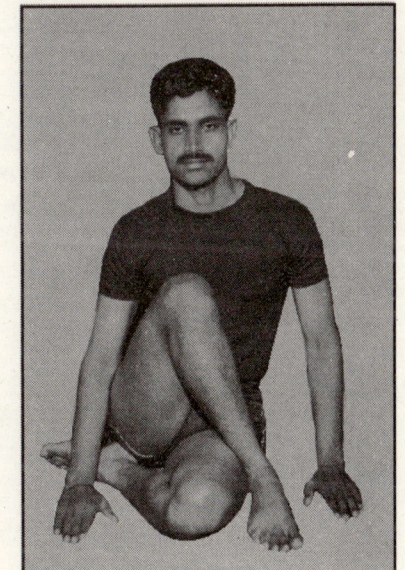

Fig. 41.0 : Front view

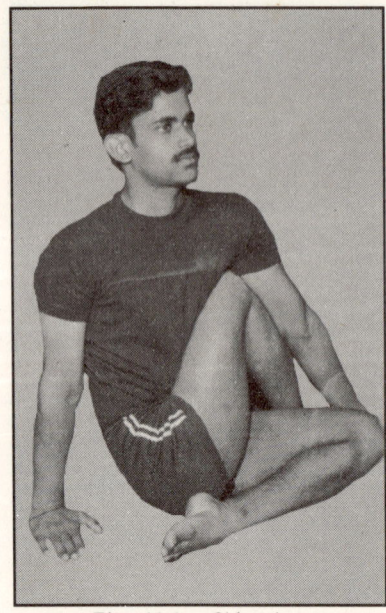
Fig. 41.1 : Side view

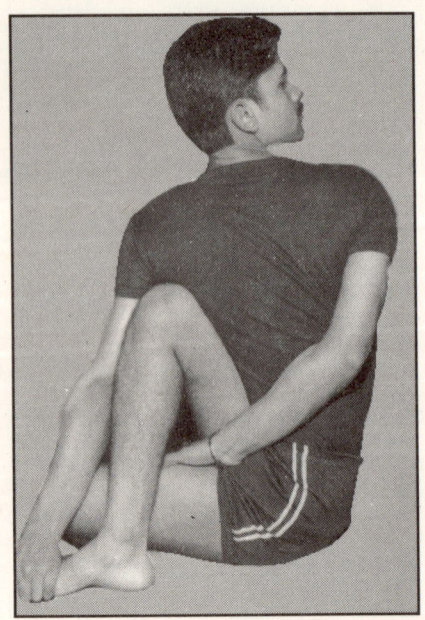
Fig. 41.2 : Back view

6. Exhale slowly and start lowering the hands and the legs in order to resume the normal position.

Precaution: Utmost care should be taken not to force the elbows too much and the spinal twist can be done slowly.

Therapeutic Advantages

1. This exercise gives strength to the thighs, shoulders, and abdominal muscles.
2. This exercise is recommended for those who are suffering from gastric complaints and stomach disorder.
3. This exercise reduces pains in the region of hips.
4. Effectively cures back pain.
5. Reduces the fat in the waist region and also tones up the kidney.

B. Purna Matsyendrasana: "Purna" means full or complete. Matsyendra as explained earlier is one of the founders of Hatha Vidhya. This is the complete and final posture of Matsyendrasana.

Technique

1. Sit on the ground and stretch the legs forward.
2. Flex the left knee and place the left foot at the root of right thigh. The heel

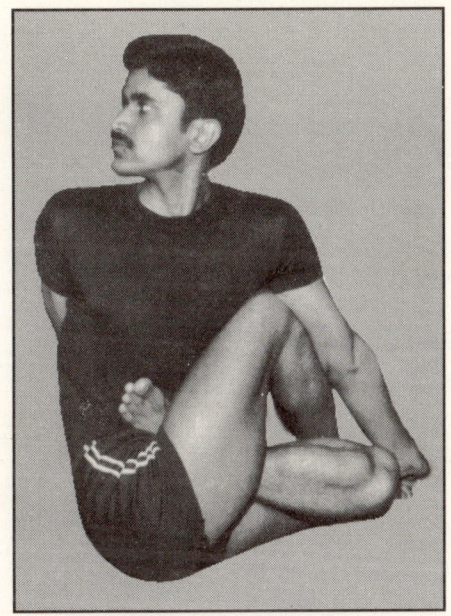
Fig. 41.3 : Front view

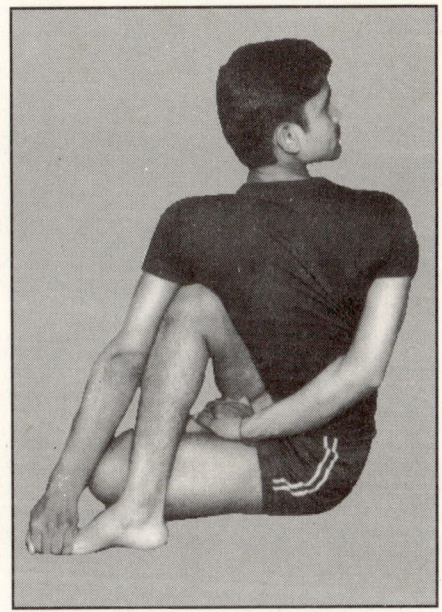
Fig. 41.4 : Back view

    should press against left navel region. Bend right knee up and bring it near the chest.
3. Exhale slowly, twist the trunk towards right, swinging the right arm from the shoulder and catch the left ankle with the right hand in the back.
4. Lift the right foot near the left thigh and place it on the ground by the outer side of the left knee.
5. Exhale, slowly turn the trunk towards right in order to bring left shoulder over the right knee and catch right foot with the left hand. (refer Fig. 41.3 and 41.4).
6. Hold in this position for about 15 to 20 seconds with the deep breathing.
7. First release the left foot and then release the grip and slowly come back to the normal position.
8. Repeat the same process on the other side also.

Therapeutic Advantages

The therapeutic uses are similar to Ardha Matsyendrasana.

42. GOMUKHASANA: (The Cow-Head Posture)

Technique

1. Sit on the ground and stretch the legs forward.

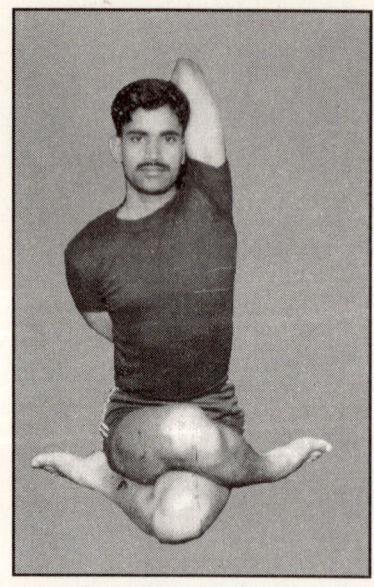

Fig. 42.0 : Front view

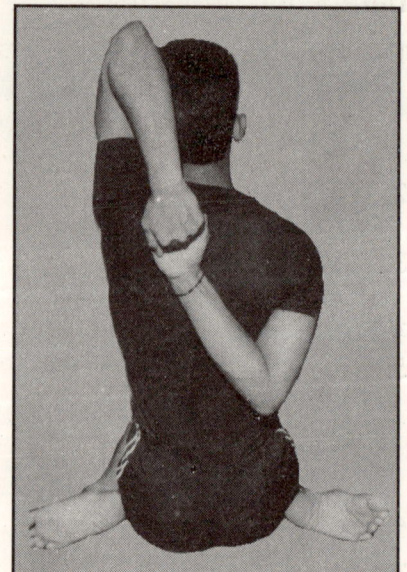

Fig. 42.1 : Back view

2. Fold the left knee back and sit on the left foot. Raise the right leg and place right thigh over the left one.
3. Slowly bring left arm to the back. Slowly take the right arm in order to make a lock as shown in the Fig. 42.0 and 42.1.

Therapeutic Advantages

1. This exercise helps to cure all the joint pains of the body.
2. This exercise gives much stretch to the hands and legs, and hence it is recommended for sportsmen.
3. By practising this exercise, the finger joints, wrists and shoulder become flexible so it is recommended for artists and craftsmen.
4. The pain in the region of shoulder and back is cured.

43. USHTRASANA: (Camel Posture)

Technique

1. Sit in Vajrasana (as in Fig 22.0).
2. Exhale slowly and get up and place the right palm over right heel and left palm over the left heel. The back should be straight.
3. Keep the neck stretched back (refer Fig. 43.0).
4. Stay in this position for about 30 seconds with normal breathing.
5. Release the hands slowly one by one and resume the normal position.

Therapeutic Advantages

1. This asana gives more exercise to the shoulder and to the back, hence it helps to cure stiffness in the back and shoulder pain.
2. This exercise helps to increase memory power and concentration.
3. This exercise helps to reduce thirst and strain of the body
4. Helps to strengthen spinal column.
5. Helps to cure kidney disorders.

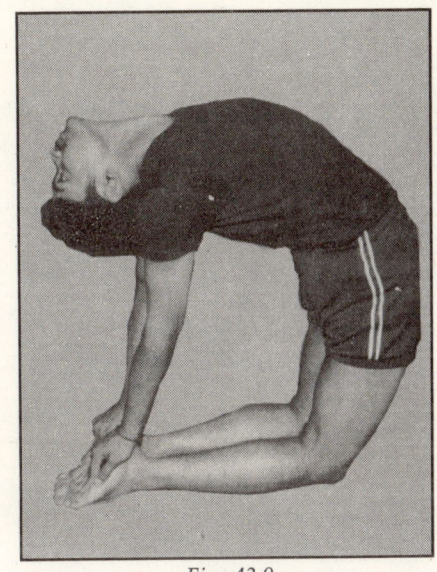

Fig. 43.0

44. LAGHU VAJRASANA

Technique

1. Sit in Vajrasana (refer Fig. 22.0)
2. Hold the knees firmly with the hands and bend backward slowly so that the crown of the hand rests on the feet (refer Fig. 44.0).
3. Stay for few seconds in this position. Exhale slowly and raise the hands and the trunk in order to resume back Vajrasana position.

Therapeutic Advantages

1. In this exercise spinal nerves are stretched so that the spinal problems, slipped disc are cured effectively.
2. This is a very good exercise for the abdomen. Performing this exercise eliminates all the abdominal diseases.
3. Since the shoulder is stretched, the shoulder pain, leg pain and other joints pain are cured.

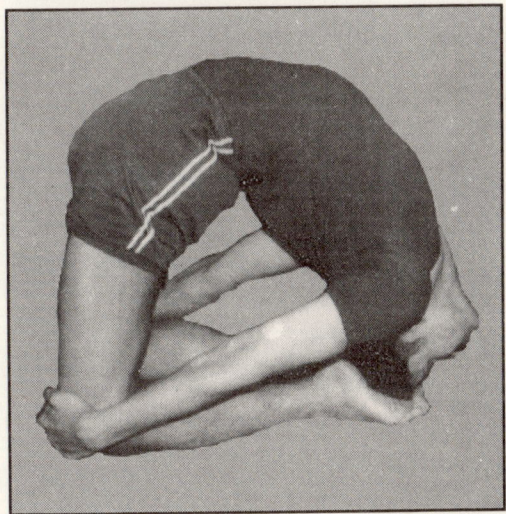

Fig. 44.0

45. KURMASANA: (The Tortoise Posture)

Technique

1. Sit on the floor and stretch the legs forward.
2. Widen the legs about a foot and a half.
3. By bending the knees, insert both the arms and stretch them straight outside (refer Fig. 45.0).
4. Rest the shoulders on the floor and keep the palms on the ground.
5. Exhale slowly and bend the trunk so that the chin should touch the floor. The legs, arms and back should be straight.
6. Stay in this position for about 30 to 40 seconds.
7. Inhale slowly, lift the head, release the hands and feet and then come back to the normal position.

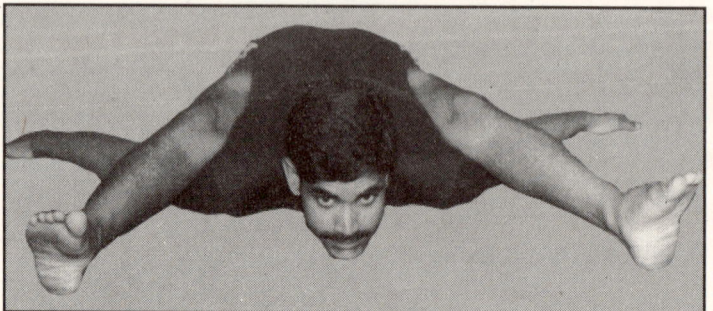

Fig. 45.0

Therapeutic Advantages

1. This yogic exercise is considered as an important spiritual discipline of yoga as it develops concentration and equilibrium. Practising this exercise develops concentration and tones up the nervous system of the body so that it reduces anxiety, anger and depression.
2. This exercise cures back pain and tones up spinal and nervous system.
3. This exercise provides good shape and beautification to the body.

46. UPAVISTA KONASANA: (Long Leg Stretch Exercise)

Technique

1. Sit on the ground and stretch the legs forward.
2. Move the legs towards both the sides and slowly widen so that they are in a straight line.
3. Stretch both hands and hold the big toes (as shown in the Fig. 46.0). Exhale and bend forward so that the chin should touch the ground.
4. Hold in this position for about 20 seconds with normal breathing.
5. Inhale slowly, raise the trunk off from the floor and release the hands and resume the normal position.

Therapeutic Advantages

1. This exercise is recommended to ladies, because it regulates menstrual flow and stimulates the ovaries.
2. This provides enough strength to legs and shoulders and hence more particularly this is beneficial for athletes and sportsmen.
3. This exercise helps to increase the height and also gives good shape to the body.
4. Most suitable for those suffering from Hernia.

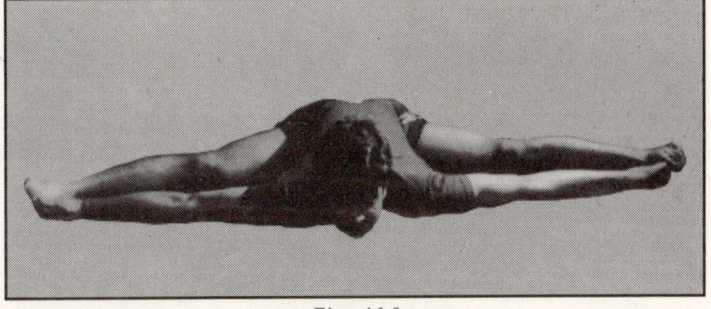

Fig. 46.0

47. NAVASANA: (Boat Posture)

Technique

1. Sit on the ground and stretch the legs forward.
2. Place the hands on the side of the body.
3. Raise the legs and thighs from the ground and simultaneously raise both the hands, so that the legs and hands are horizontal.
4. The balance should be maintained on the buttocks and no part of the body except buttock should be on the floor (refer Fig. 47.0).
5. Stay in this posture for a few seconds with normal breathing.

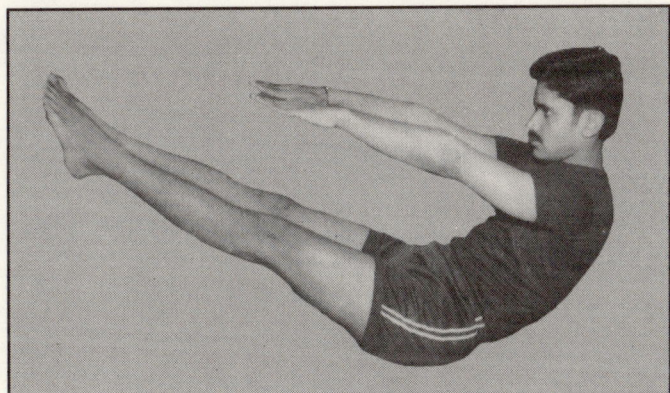

Fig. 47.0

Note: Though most of the benefits are similar to janu shirshasana, this exercise particularly helps to cure backache and nervous problem.

48. ANGUSTASANA: (Finger Balancing Posture)

In this exercise the entire body balance rests on the fingers and hence initially one can find it difficult to control the balance. With constant practice one can definitely perform this exercise effectively.

Technique

1. Sit on the ground and stretch the legs forward and keep them straight.
2. Place the hands on the ground near the thigh portion. Exhale slowly, raise the legs so that they are horizontal to the ground.
3. Ensure that the entire body balance is on the fingers (refer fig. 64.0).
4. Hold in this position for few seconds. Inhaling slowly, release the fingers and slowly bring down the legs to come back to the normal position.

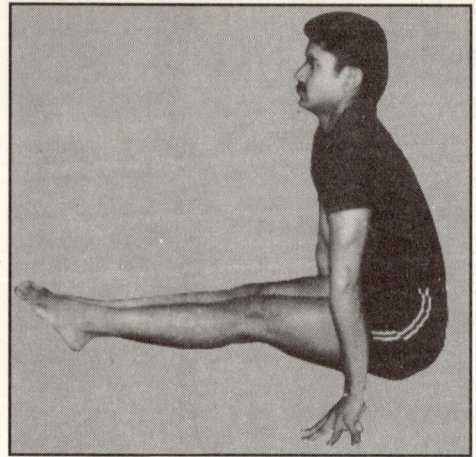

Fig. 48.0

Therapeutic Advantages

1. This exercise has a nourishing effect on the hands, fingers, the legs and the shoulders. Very effective for artists and sportsmen.
2. Cures joints and arthritic pain and abdominal disorders.

49. KANDASANA

Kanda is 12 inches above the anus and extends four inches on both the sides.

Technique

1. Sit on the ground, stretching the legs towards both the sides. With the help of hands place the feet towards the trunk (refer Fig. 49.0).
2. Hold in this position for few seconds. Release the legs slowly.

Therapeutic Advantages

1. This exercise provides greater benefits to the legs, thighs and muscles below

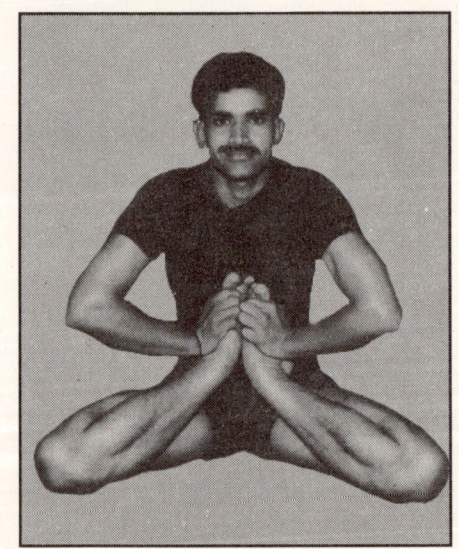

Fig. 49.0

the navel region. Cures stiffness in the hips and also joint pains in the region of legs.
2. Practising this exercise gives sexual vigour.

50. BAKASANA: (The Crane Posture)

Technique

1. Join the legs together. Place the palm on the ground and bend the trunk. The shoulder should touch the knees (refer Fig. 50.0).
2. Raise the legs above slowly, lift the head and keep the hands straight (refer Fig. 50.0).
3. Stay in this position for a few seconds and then slowly release the legs in order to come back to the original position.

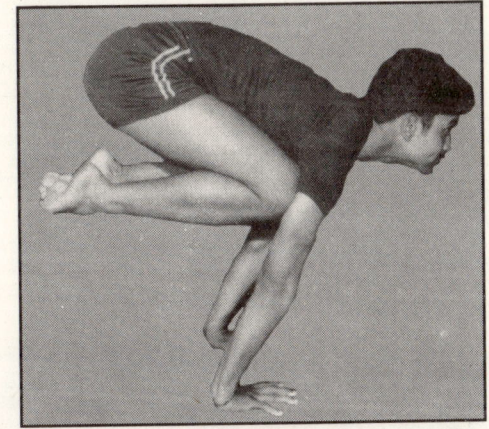

Fig. 50.0

Therapeutic Advantages

This exercise gives enough strength to the shoulders and also is a good exercise for the lower part of the belly. It cures abdominal disorders and eliminates the accumulated fat in the region of the abdomen.

51. MULABANDASANA

Technique

1. Sit in Baddha Konasana (refer Fig. 26.0)
2. Place the hands in between the thighs and hold the feet as shown in picture (refer Fig. 51.0).
3. Join the sole and then slowly raise the heels. Place the toes on the ground and drag the feet near to the perineum and place the palm near the back of the hips (refer Fig. 51.1).
4. Slowly raise the body above the floor with help of the hands and move the hips forward. Simultaneously turn

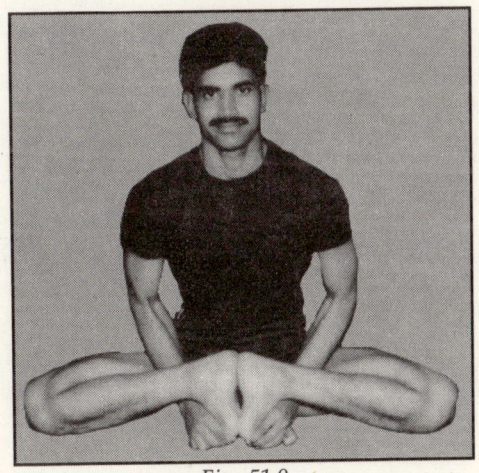

Fig. 51.0

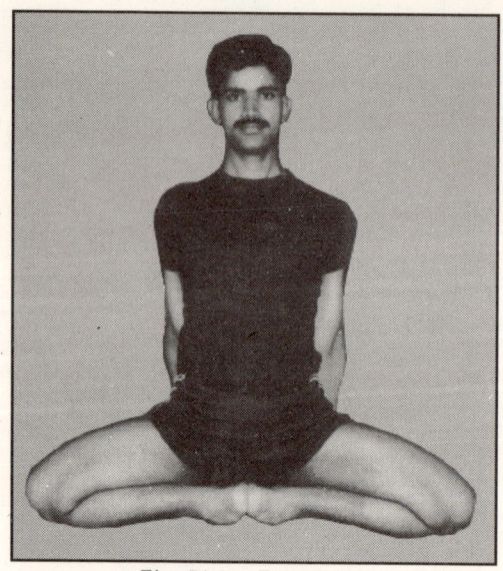

Fig. 51.1 : Front view

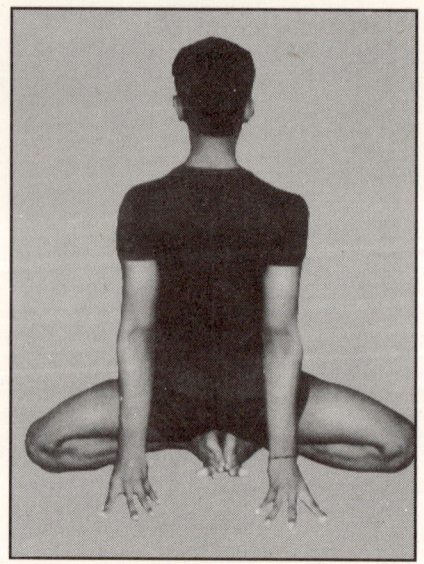

Fig. 51.2 : Back view

the feet and also the knees in order to push the heels forward (refer Figs. 51.1 and 51.2).
5. Hold in this position for a few seconds with deep breathing.

Therapeutic Advantages

1. This exercise has psychological impact which controls mind and body. Persons emotionally disturbed and those who are suffering from depression will certainly get benefited by practising this exercise.
2. This exercise checks excessive sexual desire and controls human energy and vigour.
3. It cures stiffness and pains in the region of knees, thighs, shoulders and back.

52. SAMAKONASANA: (Straight Angle Posture)

Technique

1. Sit on the ground and stretch the legs forward. The legs should be straight and be rested on the ground.
2. Slowly stretch the legs sideways so that it should form a straight line. Keep the body straight (refer Fig. 52).
3. Stay in this posture for few seconds and then slowly bring back the legs to the normal position.

Therapeutic Advantages

1. This exercise provides strength to the hip joints, and cures pain in that region.
2. The spinal problems will be cured. In this exercise the legs are stretched to the maximum extent. It helps to attain height for growing children.

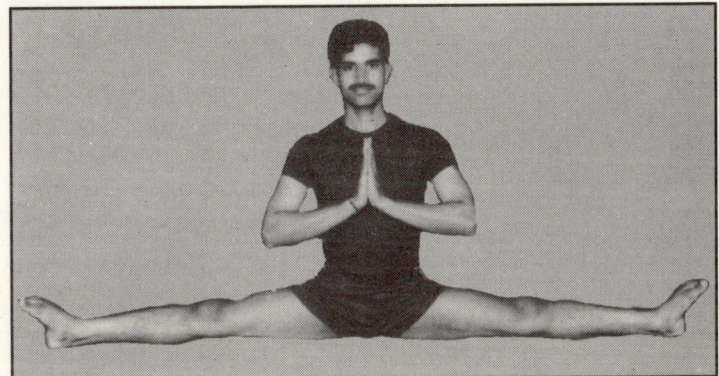

Fig. 52.0

53. TITTIBHASANA: (Insect Posture)

Technique

1. Stand straight and stretch the hands above the head.
2. Exhale slowly, bend forward and then place the palms on the floor by the sides of the hips.
3. Supporting the palm firmly, slowly lift both the legs so that it should touch the shoulder (refer Fig. 53.0). The body and knees should be straight and well stretched.

Therapeutic Advantages

1. This is one of the key exercises to cure chronic back pain and it is recommended for working professionals, executives suffering from severe back pain.
2. In this exercise the lower part of the stomach, thighs, and shoulders are stretched extensively and hence joints pain will be cured.
3. In this exercise the entire body is balanced on the palms. This is a very good exercise for hands and

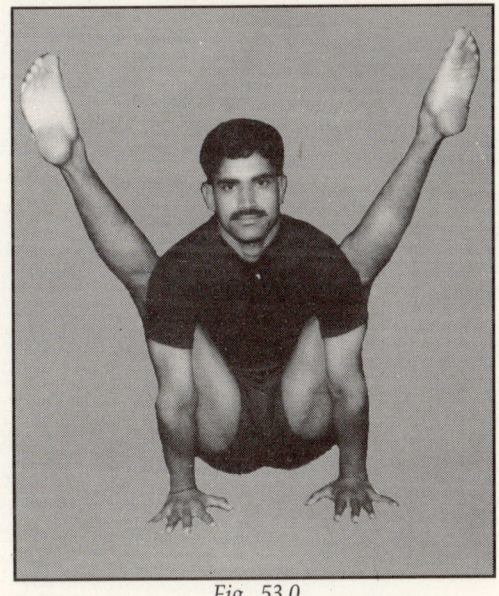

Fig. 53.0

shoulders as well as the legs. Hence this exercise is most beneficial to athletes and players.

54. URDHWAMUKHA TITTIBHASANA

'Urdhwa' means 'upward'. 'Tittibha' means an 'insect'. This exercise is performed, by keeping the face upward as explained below.

Technique

1. Stand as in Fig. 1.0.
2. Spread the legs apart sideways for about one and half to two feet. Exhale slowly, bend the trunk forward. Insert the head in between the legs at knee position. Stretch the hands towards the back and make a lock (as shown in Fig. 54.0).
3. Hold in this position for about 15 to 20 seconds with deep and even breathing.
4. Release the interlock first and slowly come back to the normal position.

Therapeutic Advantages

1. Though most of the therapeutic uses are similar to Tittibhasana, here in this exercise it provides good body balance, nourishment to the legs and shoulders.
2. This exercise provides mental equilibrium and concentration of mind.

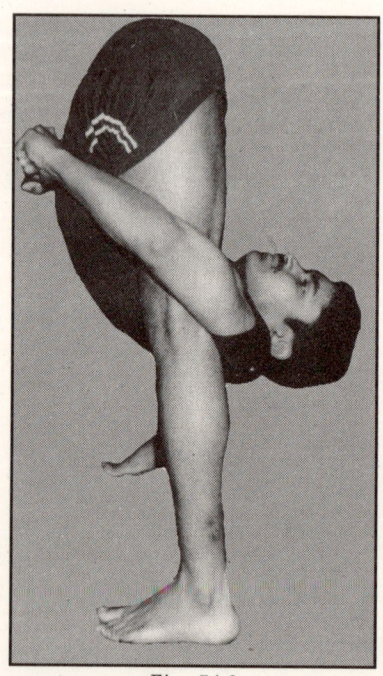

Fig. 54.0

55. VIPARITHA KARNI: (The Inverted Posture)

In Hatha yoga deepika the Viparitha karni is considered as Mudra and not an asana. In usual practice though we are not differentiating too much between the terms Asana and Mudra, but in Hatha Yoga, the dandas and mudra are used distinctively. Even in Sanskrit literature the word Asana, Bandha and Mudra are used in the same sense. In Sanskrit viparitha means 'inverted', 'karni' means 'action'. The essence of viparitha karni is "Keeping the head down and legs above the head." Practising this exercise helps to conveniently perform Sarvangasana.

Technique

1. Lie down on the floor in a complete relaxed position.
2. Exhale slowly and raise the legs and hips with the support of arms.
3. Hold the hips with the hands (refer Fig. 55.0).
4. Hold in this pose for a few seconds and breathe normally.
5. Inhale slowly and lower the legs towards the ground and return to the relaxed position.
6. Continue the process 2 to 3 times.

Precaution: Those who are suffering from high blood pressure and weak heart should not practise this exercise without prior consultation with the yoga master.

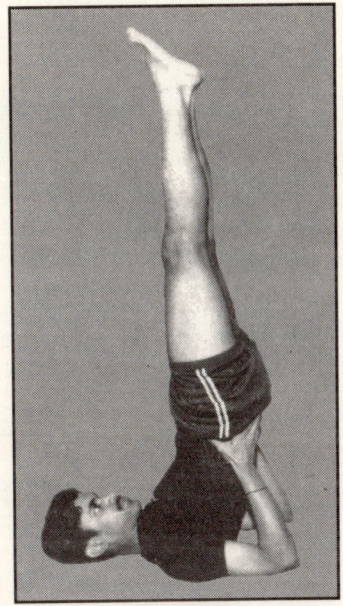

Fig. 55.0

Therapeutic Advantages

1. This helps to control the body weight.
2. Helps to provide good blood circulation to the body, which helps to cure breathing problems, activating the nerve centres of the brain.
3. Practising this exercise provides better blood flow to the neck, throat and head. The problems in the region of neck, throat, and head are cured.
4. This exercise serves as an aid to increase the facial beauty because good circulation of blood gives tenderness to the face and cheek.

56. SARVANGASANA: (Shoulder Stand Posture)

The name itself suggests that in this exercise the entire body is activated. Because of this reason it is termed as Sarvangasana. Those who are acquainted with Viparitha karni can easily perform this exercise. The precautions explained in viparitha karni hold well for this exercise also. This is one of the important yogic practices in Hatha yoga. This is much more strenuous and difficult as compared to viparitha karni.

Technique

1. Resume the posture of viparitha karni (refer Fig. 55.0) and then slowly raise the hips still higher so that the entire back is perpendicular to the ground and the chin is pressed against the chest. Legs should be straight. (refer Fig. 56.0).
2. Few people experience watering in the eyes. In such cases, they are advised

to practise by closing eyes. Hold for about a minute and slowly bend the legs down.
3. Relax completely for about a minute.

Precaution: It is to be done once only. Those who are suffering from high blood pressure and heart ailment should start practice only with the consultation of the yoga master.

Therapeutic Advantages:

Performing this exercise gives several benefits since the entire body is in action. The entire body is activated and the complete body system is toned up.

1. Those who are suffering from eyesight defects, this exercise helps considerably.
2. Due to increased supply of blood to the brain the students must perform this exercise which gives increased memory power and concentration.
3. The problems in the area of thyroid glands are cured.
4. The pains in the region of leg and diseases of the nervous system are eliminated.
5. Arrests premature aging, gives youthfulness and vigour and serves as a beautification tool.
6. This is the best exercise for those who are suffering from ovarian problems. Ensures the good functioning of sexual and reproductive organs. People suffering from impotency are advised to practise this exercise without fail.
7. Excutive's stress is cured. Practising this exercise relieves anxiety due to stress.
8. Helps to cure insomnia and mental depression.
9. It helps to cure constipation, gastric disorders and abdominal problems.

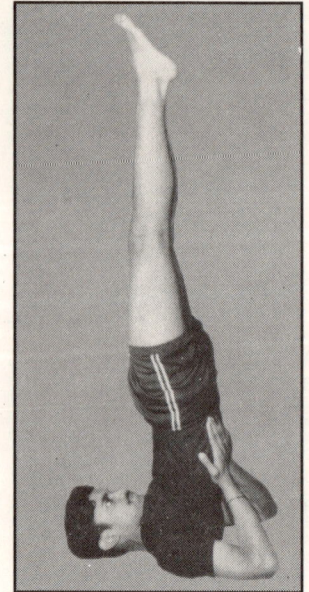

Fig. 56.0

57. HALASANA: (The Plough Posture)

It is an extension of viparitha karni and is considered as one of the best Hatha yoga systems.

Technique

1. Start with Sarvangasana posture (refer Fig. 56.0).
2. Stretch the hands back on the floor with the palm touching the ground. Move the trunk upwards so that toes rest on the floor (refer Fig. 57.0). Chin

is to be pressed against chest.
3. Hold for 15 to 20 seconds with normal breathing.
4. Return back slowly to the normal position.
5. Repeat the process only twice.

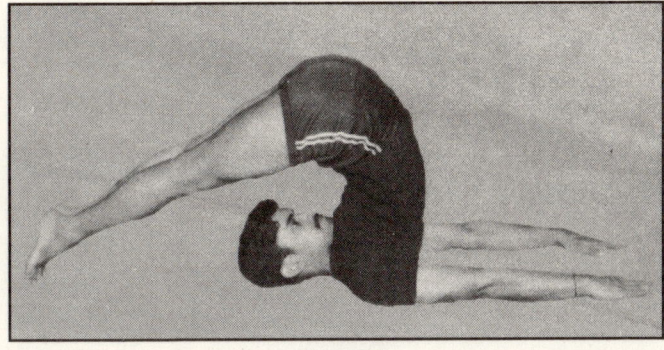
Fig. 57.0

Precaution: Those who are suffering from stiffness in spinal column or long illness are advised to practise this asana under the supervision of yoga teacher.

Therapeutic Advantages

1. Most beneficial exercise for the spinal column.
2. It helps to strengthen the spinal cord, which gets maximum stretch and hence all the disorders will be rectified.
3. Abdominal muscles are stretched and defect in that region will be cured. Ensures good digestion and appetite. Practising this exercise helps to give physical beauty, youthfulness and good shape to the body.
4. Activates the glandular systems and helps to cure menstrual disorder.
5. It reduces the excess fat in the region of hips and waist.
6. Provides youthfulness to the face and to the body.
7. It nourishes the sexual organ and provides sexual power and vigour. Strengthens the weak sex glands.

58. SUPTHA KONASANA

Though it is similar to Halasana there is a little variation in this exercise.

Technique

1. Perform Halasana (Fig. 57.0).
2. From Halasana stretch the legs outwards straight (as shown in the Fig. 58.0). Keep the trunk up and straight.

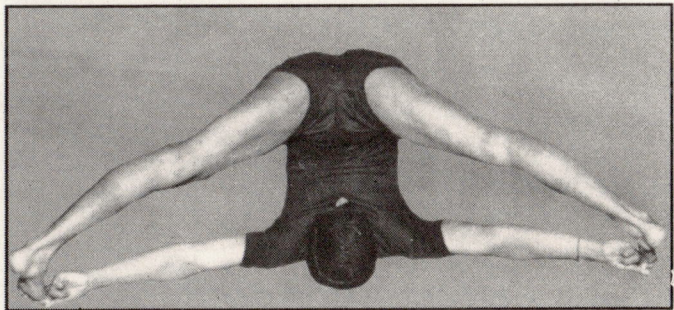
Fig. 58.0

3. Hold the right toe with right hand and left toe with the left hand.
4. Hold for about 30 seconds with normal breathing.

Therapeutic Advantages

1. Gives enough strength to the legs and hands. The pain in the region of shoulders, knees, thighs, and ankles are cured. Recommended to athletes and sports people.
2. It increases the body height for growing children.
3. Abdominal organs are toned up and diseases in those parts are cured.

59. SETU BANDA SARVANGASANA: (Bridge Posture)

Technique

1. First perform Viparitha karni (refer Fig. 55.0).
2. Rest the palms firmly on the back and lift the hips and waist upward retaining shoulders and feet on the floor. Stretch the legs and keep them together (Fig. 59.0).
3. While doing the process, it forms a bridge, the weight lies on elbows and wrists.
4. Fig. 59.1 refers to Ekapada Setubanda Sarvangasana. In this exercise though it is similar to setubanda sarvangasana, after performing Setubanda Sarvangasana exhale slowly and lift right leg up to a perpendicular level.
5. Hold for about 30 seconds with normal breathing.
6. Release the palms slowly and back to the normal position.

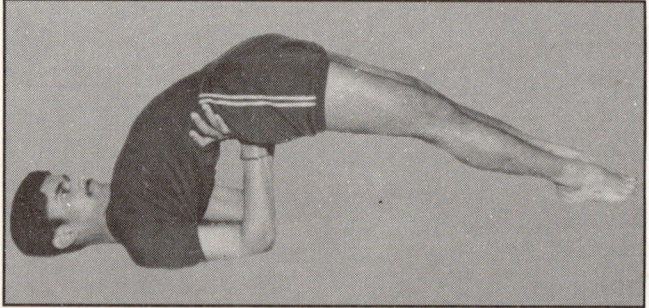

Fig. 59.0

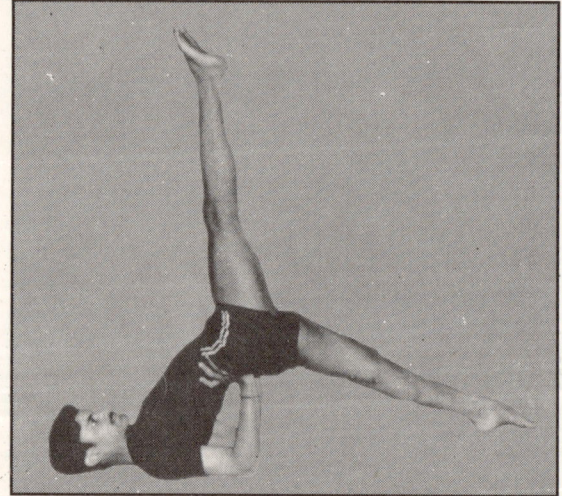

Fig. 59.1

Therapeutic Advantages

1. Cures pain in the region of neck, shoulder, knees and thighs.

2. Gives nourishing effect to spinal cord and also the neck pain is cured completely.
3. Cures kidney problems and removes the fat in the region of hips and stomach.
4. Helps to nourish the entire nervous system of the body.
5. Helps to cure gastric trouble and respiratory disorders.

60. JATHARA PARIVARTHANASANA: (Stomach Rolling Posture)

Technique

1. Lie flat on the ground and stretch the arms towards both the sides. Keep the shoulders straight.
2. Exhale slowly, raise both the legs together so that they should be perpendicular to the ground (refer Fig. 60.0).
3. Hold in this position for few seconds. Exhale, slowly move both the legs sideways so that the toes must touch the ground. Ensure to keep the back straight and on the floor (refer Fig. 60.1).
4. Hold in this position for few seconds.
5. Practise on the other side with the same process.

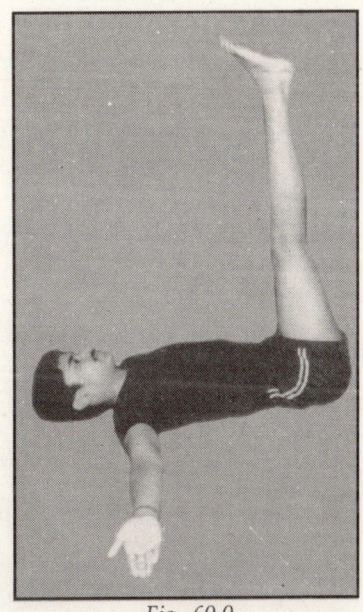

Fig. 60.0

Therapeutic Advantages

1. As the name suggests, this exercise helps to stimulate the stomach region and also helps to reduce excess fat in that region.
2. This is the most beneficial exercise for those who are suffering from stomach pain, indigestion, and gastritis and stomach disorders.
3. This exercise removes the problem in the area of liver, spleen and pancreas.
4. This help to cure back pain and pain in the region of hip.

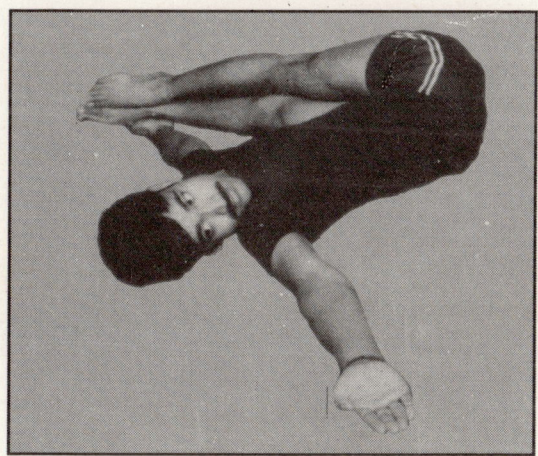

Fig. 60.1

61. HANUMANASANA

This asana is dedicated to Lord Anjunaya because of its significance and spiritual values. Practising this exercise helps to provide the courage, strength and power of Lord Hanuman. Hence it has significant importance in yogic science.

Technique

1. Sit on the ground. Place the palms on either side of the body.
2. Slowly lift the knees up. Bring the right leg forward and left leg back. The leg should be straight, stretched and horizontal to the ground. The entire body support should lie on the palms (refer Fig. 61.0). When the balance is attained slowly remove the palm from the ground and perform namaskar.
3. Ensure that back and the entire body is straight and firm.
4. Stay in this posture for about 10 to 20 seconds with even breathing.

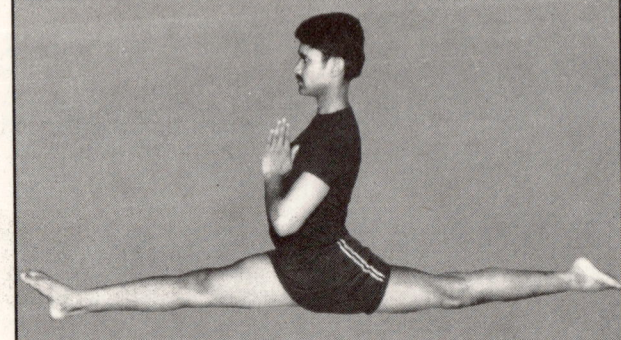

Fig. 61.0

Therapeutic Advantages

1. In this asana the legs are stretched very well and hence it is most suitable for athletes and sportsmen.
2. This asana is most suitable for ladies because performing this exercise helps to cure various gynaecological problems.

62. HANUMANA VALIKILYASANA

This is an advanced yogic practice of Hanumanasana. This is a difficult yogic exercise and it requires constant follow up and practice.

Technique

1. Perform Hanumanasana (refer Fig. 61.0).
2. After performing Namaskar slowly raise the hands towards the back so that hands are near the ankle region.
3. Slowly move the head and back so that the head should touch the hip region (refer Fig. 62.0).

4. Stay in this posture for about 8 to 10 seconds, with even breathing. Slowly move the head forward and release the handgrips and come back to Hanumanasana.

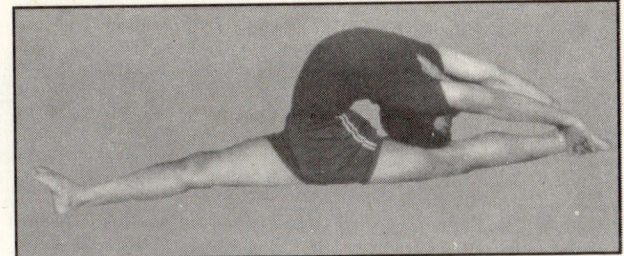
Fig. 62.0

Therapeutic Advantages

1. This asana gives enough strength and support to the legs, hands, back and the neck.
2. Most of the therapeutic advantages are similar to Hanumanasana.

63. VIBHAKTA JANUSHIRSHASANA

Vibhakta means, "separate". Janu refers to "knee" and shirsha means "the head". Here separate the legs towards opposite direction and then place the head on the knee.

Technique

1. Perform Hanumanasana (refer Fig. 61.0).
2. Raise the hands upward. Exhale slowly and bend the back so that chin touches the foot. (refer Fig. 63.0)

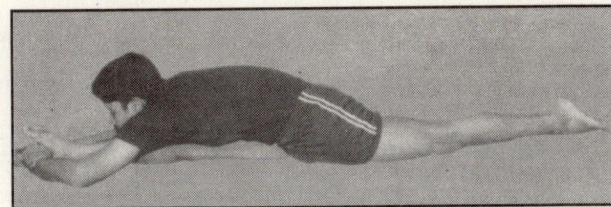
Fig. 63.0

3. Slowly moving the head towards the knee, grip the toes. The crown of the head should touch the knee (refer Fig. 63.1). Entire body should be firm and stretched.
4. Stay in this position for about 10 to 20 seconds with normal breathing.
5. Inhale slowly, raise the head above and then slowly release the handgrip in order to resume normal position.

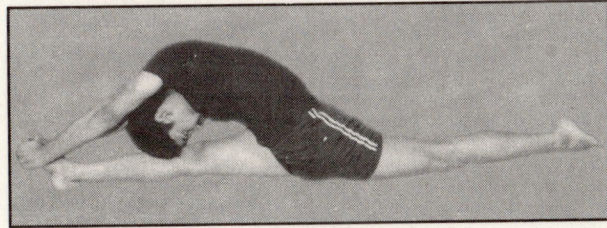
Fig. 63.1

Therapeutic Advantages

1. This exercise gives strength to the arms, legs, back and shoulders. Hence this exercise is very useful to athletes and sportsmen.
2. The joint pain, shoulder pain and back pain are cured.
3. It helps to reduce the fat in the region of stomach and hips.
4. The stomach problem and digestive disorder are eliminated.

64. EKAPADA SHIRSHASANA

Technique

1. Lie down on the floor and stretch the legs forward.
2. Bend the knees and lift the leg with the support of hands.
3. Exhale slowly, place the leg at the back of the neck portion. Lift the neck and head so that it is straight (refer Fig. 64.0).
4. Stay in this position for about 15 to 30 seconds.
5. With the support of the hands, take back the leg to the normal position. Practise this exercise alternatively for both the legs.

Caution : While placing the leg on the back of the neck and also while stretching the knees, one should perform very slowly. Otherwise in some instances sprain in the region of neck or in the region of knees will be felt.

Therapeutic Advantages

1. This is an effective exercise to cure neck and back pain.
2. It strengthens the joints in the region of knees and also gives strength to the shoulders.

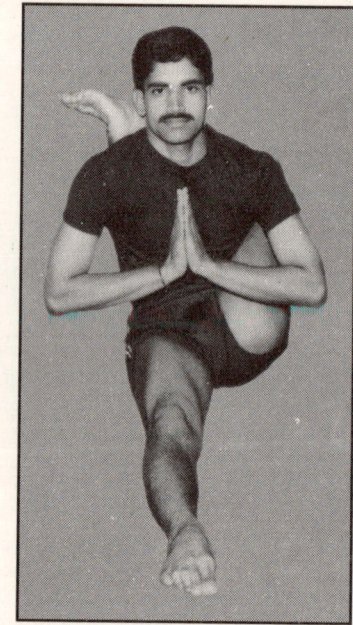

Fig. 64.0

65. CHAKORASANA: (Wing Posture)

Technique

1. Perform Ekapada Shirshasana.
2. Raise the legs so that it should be of 60° angle. The entire body balance is on fingers (refer Fig. 65.0).
3. Stay in this position for few seconds, thereafter place the legs slowly on the ground and also release the legs slowly.
4. Repeat this exercise on the other side alternatively.

Therapeutic Advantages

1. An effective exercise which gives enough strength to the shoulder and legs.
2. Cures all the abdominal disorders and also gives strength to the neck.
3. In this exercise the entire body balance rests on the fingers. This gives strength and flexibility to the fingers. Hence artists will benefit from this exercise.

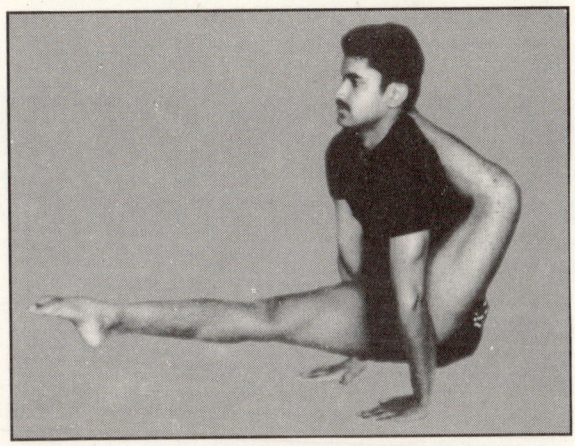

Fig. 65.0

66. OMKARASANA

This asana is most precious and having spiritual values. Chanting of **OMKARA** is believed to clean body and mind. This asana is a symbolic representation to provide spiritual, physical and mental discipline.

Technique

1. Perform Chakorasana (refer Fig. 65.0).
2. After performing Chakorasana, stretched leg should be folded and locked just below the shoulder. The entire body balance should be on the palms. The body should be straight and erect (refer Fig. 66.0).
3. Stay in this position for about 10 to 20 seconds with even breathing and slowly come back to the normal position.

Therapeutic Advantages

1. As the name itself suggests, this exercise provides physical and mental discipline. This asana not only cures physical disorders but also cures mental disorders.

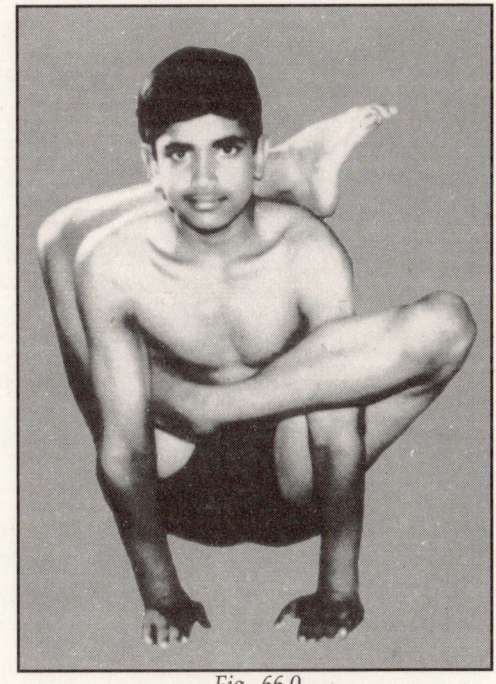

Fig. 66.0

2. This asana helps to increase memory power and mental sharpness. Most useful for children and students.
3. It provides strength to the shoulder and tones up the entire physical structure of the body.

67. DWIPADA SHIRSHASANA

In this yogic exercise both the legs are stretched and placed on the back. Those who are familiar with Ekapada Shirshasana can easily practise this exercise with little effort.

Technique

1. Start Ekapada Shirshasana, that is, place one leg behind the back of the neck.
2. Exhale slowly and lift the other leg with the support of hand and place it behind the neck.
3. Place hands on the floor and lift the hands off from the floor, so that the entire body balance is supported with the hands (refer Fig. 67.0).
4. Stay in this posture for a few seconds and release the foot locks slowly and then resume normal position.

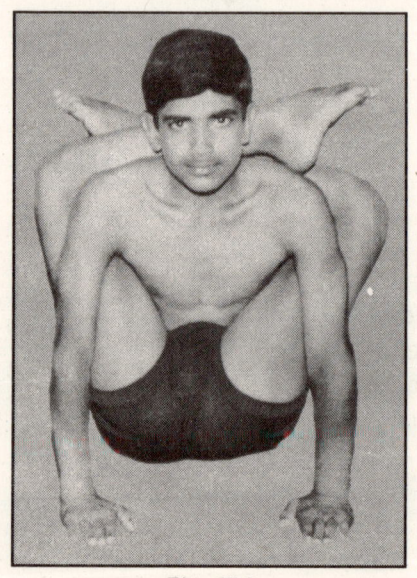

Fig. 67.0

Therapeutic Advantages

1. In this exercise the abdominal muscle and the lungs are stretched and hence it tones up all the abdominal functions and also cures lung disorders.
2. The shoulder, the neck, the legs and the back are stretched and gives good support to that entire region.
3. Though it is difficult to perform this exercise, it gives the flexibility to the entire body system. We advise yoga practioners to practise this exercise without fail.

68. DHANDAYAMAN EKAPADA SIKANDASANA: (Durvasasana)

It is also termed as Durvasasana as there is a belief that Sage Durvasa performed meditation in this posture. Whatever the belief may be, this exercise provides body and mental equilibrium.

Technique

1. Perform Ekapada Shirshasana (refer Fig. 64.0).
2. Slowly wake up, ensure the leg is straight (refer Fig. 68.0).
3. Stay for a few seconds in this posture.
4. Practise this exercise on the other side also.

Therapeutic Advantages

1. Stimulates legs and shoulder and automatically cures leg and shoulder pain. Very effective for athletes and sportsmen.
2. Gives body equilibrium.

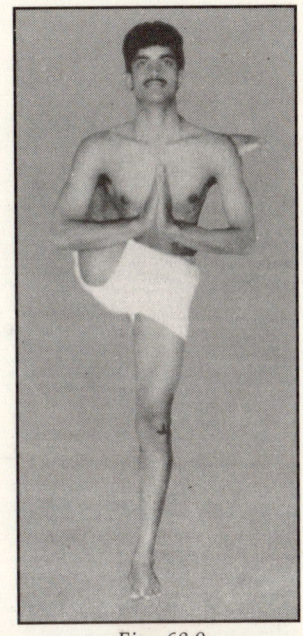
Fig. 68.0

69. YOGA NIDHRASANA

This is very important yogic exercise, which helps to provide energy to the body, and helps to control the mind. 'Nidhra' refers to a state of sleep. Yoga Nidhra is the state between sleep and wakefulness. In our epic we have read that Lord VISHNU used to sleep at the end of yoga. This symbolic representation of our epic has been given to this yogic exercise, so that it is considered as one of the important yogic exercises.

Technique

1. Lie down on ground, slowly bend both the knees so as to bring the legs over the head.
2. Exhaling slowly, bend both the legs as shown in the figure. The foot serves as pillow (refer Fig. 69.0).
3. Place the hands with grips near the hips (refer Fig. 69.0).
4. Here the legs placed behind the neck serve as pillow.
5. Ensure that the back of the upper arm is in contact with the back of the thighs.
6. Hold in this position for about 8 to 10 seconds with normal breathing.
7. Exhaling slowly, release the handgrip first and then release the leg grip.

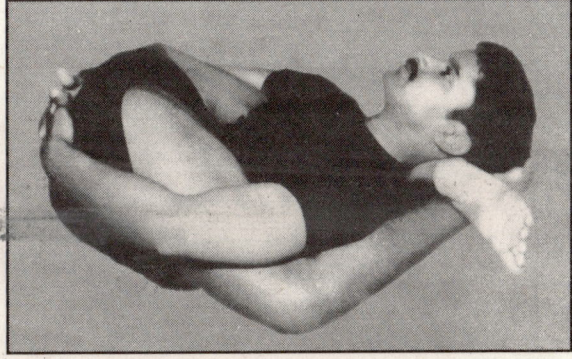
Fig. 69.0

Therapeutic Advantages

1. Practising this yogic exercise helps to get the body warmed up instantly. This exercise is advisable to athletes and sportsmen to keep the body warm immediately.
2. It involves extensive stretch of back, shoulder, legs and knees, which help to eliminate back pain, shoulder and leg pains.
3. Practising this exercise helps to cure the problem in the area of kidney, liver, spleen, intestine, gall bladder, prostates and urinary bladder.

70. BHUJANGASANA

In Sanskrit 'Bhuja' refers to 'upper arm' and 'Bhujanga' means a 'serpent'. This exercise resembles a large snake. Hence it is termed as Bhujangasana.

Technique

1. Lie down on the ground with face downward.
2. Keep the palm on the ground beside the chest.
3. Inhale slowly and raise the hand and trunk as in the shape of hood of the Cobra.
4. Hold in this position for few seconds and take normal breath (refer Fig. 70.0).
5. Exhale slowly and come back to normal position.

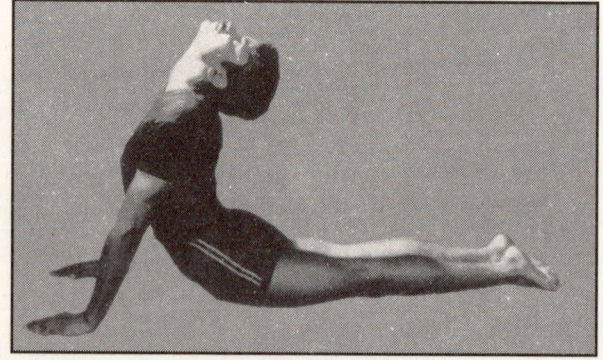

Fig. 70.0

Caution : Those who are suffering from stiffness in spinal column are advised to practise this exercise slowly.

Therapeutic Advantages

1. This exercise gives stretching to muscles of the neck, back and trunk, hence the pains in the region of neck, back and trunk are cured.
2. This exercise helps to cure slipped disc and backache.
3. The abdominal area are activated and hence the pancreas, stomach, liver, and other digestive organs will be strengthened. This cures indigestion and other abdominal disorders.
4. This exercise cures various menstrual problems.

71. PURNA BHUJANGASANA

This is the advanced posture of Bhujangasana and it is difficult to perform in the initial stage. By attaining perfection and constant practice, one can easily perform this exercise.

Technique

1. Perform Bhujangasana (refer Fig. 70.0).
2. Slowly raise the head so that the crown of the head touches the buttock region. Move the arms slowly towards the back and hold near the ankles. (refer Fig. 71.0).
3. Stay in this position for about 8 to 10 seconds with even breathing.
4. Slowly release the hand grip and also lift the head in order to come back to a normal position.

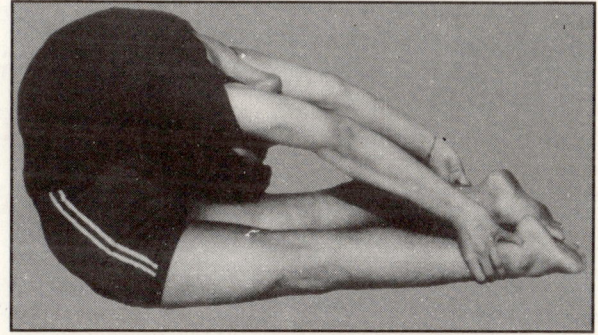

Fig. 71.0

Therapeutic Advantages

1. This exercise provides complete stretching to the muscles of neck, back and trunk. Hence the back pain, pain in the region of neck, gastric problem are effectively cured.
2. In this exercise the neck region is stretched extensively and hence the vocal tubes become clean and perfect. Hence, this exercise is particularly recommended to musicians, artists and lecturers.

72. RAJAKAPOTHASANA

'Raja' means the 'king', Rajakapothasana means the 'king of pigeons'. Here the chest, which is, pushed forward resembles the pigeon, hence this name.

Technique

1. Perform Bhujangasana (refer Fig. 70.0).
2. By exhalation lift the head and trunk upward to the maximum extent. Bend the knees and lift the feet up.
3. Move both the hands towards back, firmly hold the knees with the hands. The head should rest on the soles and heels.

4. Hold in this position for about 10 to 15 seconds.
5. Release the hands first and place the palms in front on the floor. Thereafter slowly rest the chest on the floor and relax.

Therapeutic Advantages

1. In this exercise the lumbar region of the spine are stretched well and hence the problems in those regions will be effectively cured.
2. The neck and shoulder pain is relieved.
3. Due to increased blood circulation in the area of thyroids, parathyroid and adrenal glands, the problem in those areas is cured.
4. As the abdominal organs are pressed on the floor while performing this exercise, all the abdominal problems are cured.

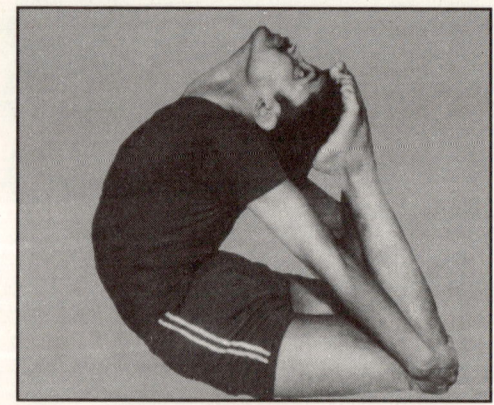

Fig. 72.0

73. EKAPADA RAJAKAPOTHASANA

Technique

1. Perform Hanumanasana (refer Fig. 61.0).
2. Stretch the chest forward and push the head back as much as possible. Bend the left knee and place it near the head. The knee should be perpendicular.
3. By exhalation move the left arm over the head and grip the left foot. Take few breaths. Start exhalation and place the right arm over the head and catch the left foot with right hand.(refer Fig. 73.0).
4. Stay in this position for about 8 to 10 seconds and then slowly release the grip. Finally come back to Hanumanasana.

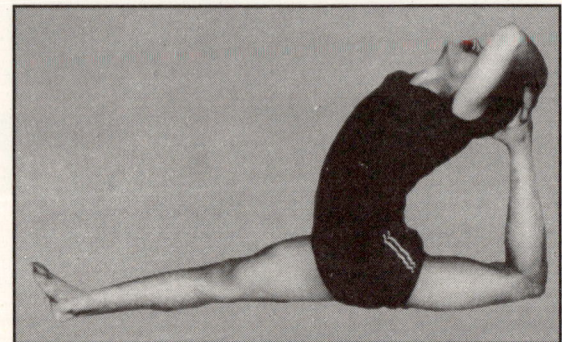

Fig. 73.0

Therapeutic Advantages

1. In this exercise the neck and shoulder muscle are fully exercised. Also strengthen the thighs, legs and the ankles, hence it is recommended for athletes and sportsmen.

2. This exercise is also recommended for growing children in order to attain height and personality.
3. This exercise helps to eliminate urinary disorders and also checks sexual diseases.
4. Due to increase of blood circulation to thyroids, parathyroid, and adrenal glands, the disorders in those region are effectively cured.
5. This exercise also helps to cure backache and spinal problems.

74. SHALABHASANA: (Locist Posture)

There are two types of exercises in Shalabhasana.
    A. Ekapada Shalabhasana
    B. Dwipada Shalabhasana

Technique

1. Lie down on the floor with the face downwards.
2. Stretch the legs so that the toes are flat down on the ground. The whole body should be straight and stiff.
3. Stretch the arms and place the thumbs freely on the ground.
4. Inhale slowly, raise the left leg slowly as high as possible. (refer Fig. 74.0). This exercise is termed as Ardha Shalabhasana and those who feel difficult to raise both the legs are advised to perform this exercise alternatively for both the legs. Stay for about 30 seconds on each side. Slowly bring down the legs and release.

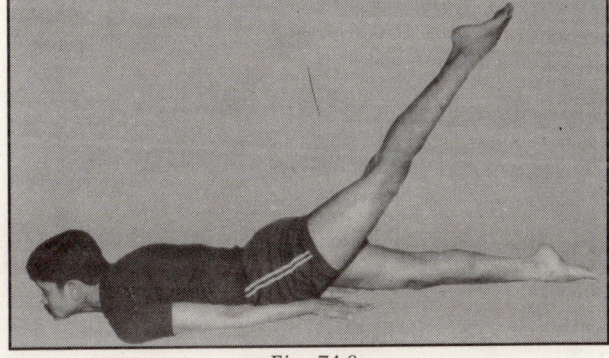
Fig. 74.0

5. In Dwipada Shalabhasana try to raise both the legs slowly to the possible extent as shown in the posture. (refer Fig. 74.1).
6. Hold few seconds with normal breathing.
7. Exhale slowly and bring the legs down towards the ground and relax.

Suggestion: It is advised to practise Ardha Shalabhasana first which helps to perform Shalabhasana once practice is continued for some time.

Therapeutic Advantages

1. This exercise helps to cure diabetes and prostate gland problems.

2. This exercise gives good effect to the whole body and helps to tone up spine, lungs, chest, neck and shoulder.
3. This cures various abdominal troubles including problems in the area of kidneys, liver, and pancreas.

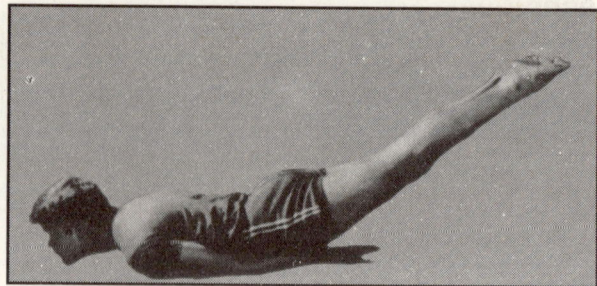

Fig. 74.1

4. It cures pains in the region of thighs and legs and hence it is recommended for athletes and sportsmen.
5. This exercise helps to cure chronic constipation.

(The therapeutic use of Ardha Shalabhasana is similar to Shalabhasana as explained above.)

75. SHALABHASANA II

This is an advanced exercise of Shalabhasana. The simplest form starts with Ekapada Shalabhasana and once the simplest form is practised well, one can try this advanced posture of Shalabhasana. In the initial stage one can find it difficult to perform and attain the balance. Regular practice can help to perform this exercise quite easily.

Technique

1. Perform Shalabhasana (refer Fig. 74.1).
2. Slowly lift the body upwards so that the entire body balance lies on the shoulder and on the chin. The shoulder and the chin should touch the ground. (refer Fig. 75.0).
3. The body should be straight, erect and stretched well.
4. Hold in this position for about 8 to 10 seconds.

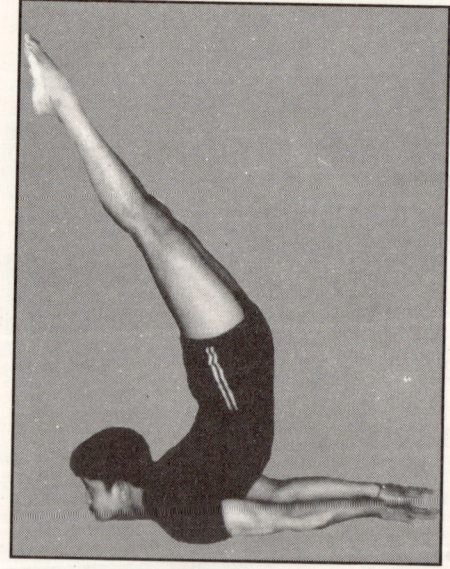

Fig. 75.0

76. PURNA SHALABHASANA

After performing Shalabhasana II one can proceed to practice the still more advanced posture of Shalabhasana explained below.

Technique

1. After staying 8 to 10 seconds in the earlier posture (refer Fig. 75.0), slowly bend the legs and the trunk so that the feet touch the crown of the head.
2. The legs and thighs should be stretched well (refer Fig. 76.0).
3. Hold in this position for 8 to 10 seconds with normal breathing.

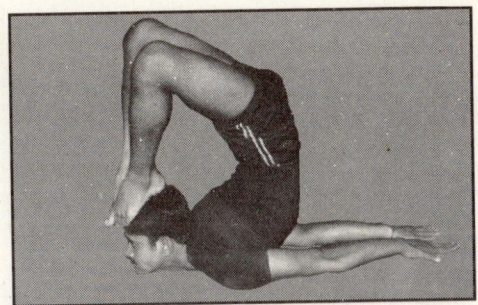
Fig. 76.0

77. VIPAREETHA SHALABHASANA

This is the most advanced and the final stage of Shalabhasana.

Technique

1. After performing Purna Shalabhasana, slowly remove the feet from the head and then slowly slide on the ground to the maximum extent

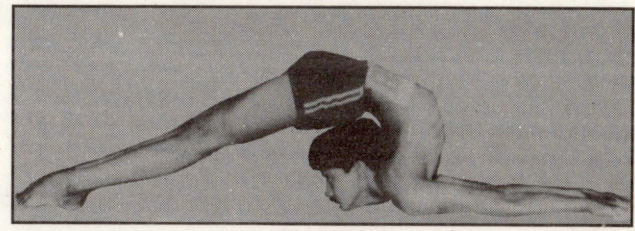
Fig. 77.0

(refer Fig. 77.0). The hip should touch the crown of the head.
2. Hold in this position for about 8 to 10 seconds with even breathing.
3. Slowly go back to the original position of Shalabhasana and then back to normal position.

Therapeutic Advantages

1. The advanced posture of Shalabhasana has several therapeutic advantages, more particularly this exercise nourishes the nervous system in Muladhara sector. So this exercise helps to increase the blood circulation in the region of pelvic plexus, hypo-gastric plexus and pharyngeal plexus.
2. This exercise helps to cure diabetes, enlarged prostate, fistula, stomach ulcer and other abdominal disorders.
3. The advanced Shalabhasana, that is, Purna and Viparitha Shalabhasana helps to provide good exercise to the eyes, particularly for central fixation.

78. MAKARASANA: (The Crocodile Posture)

Technique

1. Lie down on the floor with the face and body downward.
2. Stretch the hands above the head and ensure to stretch both the legs to a maximum extent.

3. Inhale slowly, raise both the legs and head upward (refer Fig. 78.0). Hold in this posture for a few seconds with normal breathing. The hands and legs should be stretched firmly.

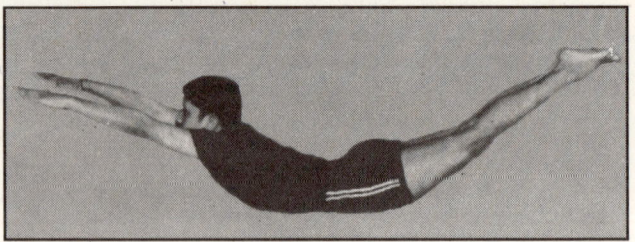
Fig. 78.0

4. Exhale slowly, lower the legs and head simultaneously.

Therapeutic Advantages

1. This posture gives maximum stretch to the back, legs and hands.
2. It cures back pain, and provides elasticity to the spinal chord.
3. As it gives maximum stretch it helps the children to grow fast and also helps to increase the height.
4. The fat in the region of hips and abdomen are effectively reduced.
5. Very good exercise to solve all the digestive problems.
6. This exercise provides maximum stretch and hence it is more suitable to athletes and sportsmen, particularly to basketball players.

79. DHANURASANA: (The Bow Posture)

Technique

1. Lie down with face and stomach downward.
2. Stretch the arms and hold the feet firmly.
3. Inhale slowly, raise the trunk and head. Continue to raise trunk, simultaneously raise the knees and head, so that the body stretches like a bow. Hold for few seconds with normal breathing. (refer Fig. 79.0).
4. Start exhaling, slowly lower the knees and the head. Repeat the exercise 2 or 3 times.
5. Release the feet, hands and relax completely.

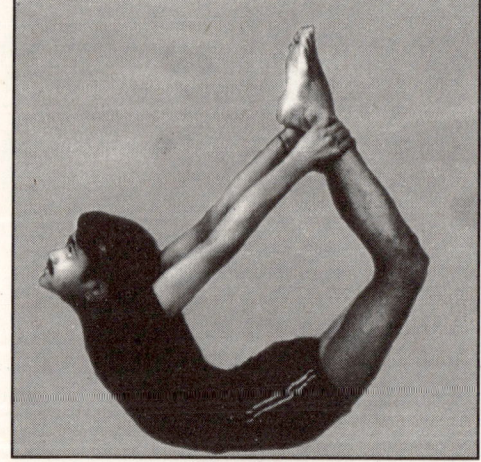
Fig. 79.0

Therapeutic Advantages

1. This exercise removes all the intestinal and the abdominal disorders. It improves the digestive system and cures constipation.

2. This exercise is recommended to those who are obese as it eliminates fat in the region of stomach, hips and thighs.
3. This is the most suitable exercise for women suffering from irregular menstruation, because in this exercise endocrine glands are toned up.
4. This exercise cures problems in the area of adrenal thyroid, parathyroid, pituitary and sexual glands.
5. It cures the disorder of joints, spinal chord and lungs. Urinary diseases, piles and gastric problems will be cured.
6. This exercise helps to provide flexibility to the spinal column and strengthens the nervous system.

80. PADANGUSTA DHANURASANA: (Finger Balance Posture)

In this asana the entire body balance rests on the fingers supported by big toe.

Technique

1. Perform Dhanurasana.
2. After attaining balance in Dhanurasana slowly raise the legs upward.
3. Slowly remove the grip from the ankle region and hold the grip with the fingers on the big toes. The legs and hands should be stretched well (refer Fig. 80.0).
4. Stay in this position for about 10 to 20 seconds, with normal breathing.
5. Slowly come back to the normal position by releasing the hand-grip.

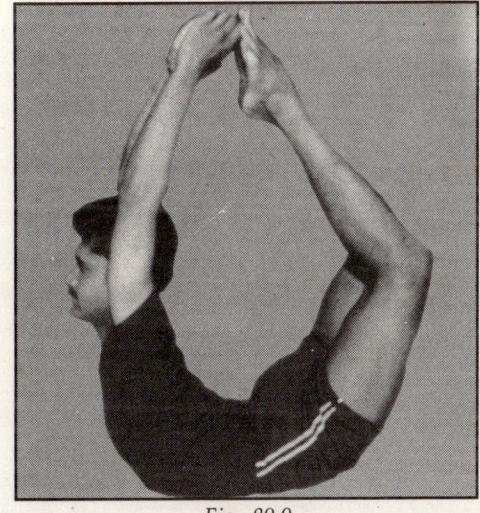
Fig. 80.0

Therapeutic Advantages

1. This asana helps to cure rheumatic and arthritic pain.
2. It cures obesity, back pain and shoulder pain.
3. It eliminates gastric problems and other digestive disorders.
4. It provides good physique and body posture.
5. It cures diabetes, asthma and bronchial disorders.

81. PURNA DHANURASANA

This is the final and the advanced posture of Dhanurasana. This exactly resembles a Dhanush (the Bow).

Technique

1. Perform Padagustha Dhanurasana.
2. After attaining the balance slowly bend the legs in the knee's region so that it is horizontal to the ground. The hand should be firm and straight (refer Fig. 81.0).

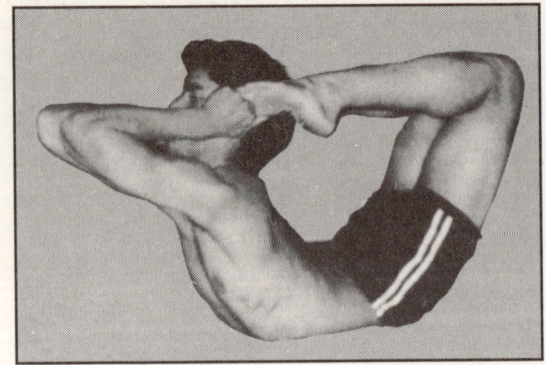

Fig. 81.0

Therapeutic Advantages:

Similar to Dhanurasana and Padangustha Dhanurasana.

82. URDHVA DHANURASANA

'Urdhva' means 'Upwards', 'Dhanu' refers to a 'bow'. This exercise can be done in two stages which is explained below.

Technique

1. Lie down with face upward, bend the knees so that the feet touch the hips.
2. Exhale, raise the back and trunk slowly as shown in the figure. The head and neck should rest on the floor (refer Fig. 82.0).
3. Hold in this posture for about 15 to 20 seconds with even breathing.
4. Slowly come back to the normal position and relax.
5. This is the first phase of Urdhva Dhanurasana. Once this exercise is well practised the following stage will be performed easily.
6. In this stage, continue to raise back and trunk so that the crown of the head should touch the ground (refer Fig. 82.1).

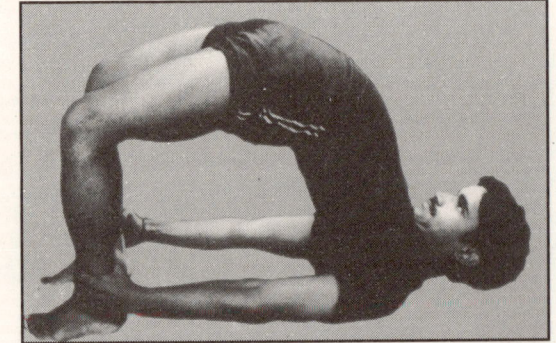

Fig. 82.0

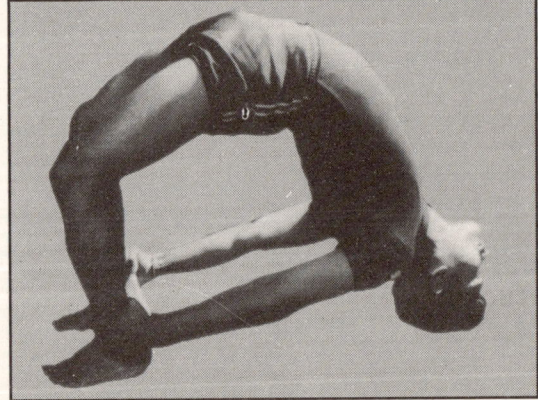

Fig. 82.1

Therapeutic Advantages

1. This exercise helps to cure back pain and also pain in the region of neck.
2. Joint pain in the region of knees and in the region of legs are cured.
3. This exercise develops concentration and control of mind.

83. AKARNA DHANURASANA

This is one of the wonderful yogic exercises, which has several benefits for the human body system.

Technique

1. Sit on the ground and stretch the legs straight forward.
2. Hold right big toe by left hand and left big toe by a right hand. Hold the big toes with the help of index and middle fingers.
3. Exhale, slowly fold the left leg at the knee's position and insert below the shoulder of the left hand. Pull the left foot up until the heel is near the right ear (refer Fig. 83.0).
4. Hold in this position for about 15 to 20 seconds with normal breathing.
5. Slowly bring down the left leg to the ground and keep both the legs stretched on the ground.
7. Repeat the exercise on the other side as explained above.

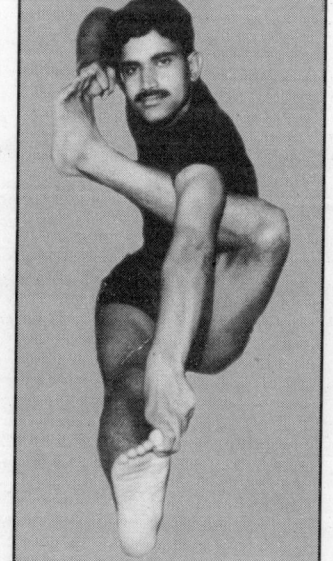

Fig. 83.0

Therapeutic Advantages

1. This exercise gives severe stretch to the muscles, hip joints and shoulders. Hence this exercise will help cure joints pain and rheumatic pains.
2. While performing this exercise the abdominal muscles are contracted which helps movement of bowels. Hence it cures all the abdominal disorders and strengthens the digestive system.

84. SHIRSHASANA: (Head Stand Posture)

Technique

1. Sit on the ground and place the forearms on the ground. Join the hands and interlock with the fingers. Place the head in middle the interlocked hand. Raise the hips and bring near the head.

2. Raise the feet slowly by bending the knees. Thereafter stretch the legs till the entire body is vertical to the ground (refer Fig. 84.0).
3. Breathe normally. Stay in this position for about 1-2 minutes.
4. To come down, bend the knees slowly and once the feet and knees touch the ground, release the hands slowly.

Precautions:
1. Those who are suffering from high blood pressure, weak heart and ear ache should not practise this exercise.
2. Shirshasana should not be practiced immediately after performing difficult yogic exercises.

Therapeutic Advantages

1. This is one of the most useful exercises to control the entire nervous system. It gives good health to all sensory organs because of better circulation of blood to the entire body system.

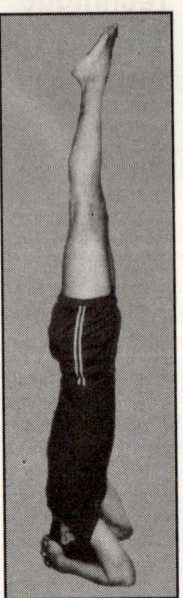

Fig. 84.0

2. Due to the handstand position there is an abundant blood circulation to brain which helps to develop good memory and concentration. It is recommended to students and school going children.
3. Entire digestive system is toned up and it cures liver problems too.
4. Most suited to athletes, sportsmen, and working professionals since this exercise provides mental concentration which is more important to these people.
5. Those who suffer from loss of sleep, memory will benefit by practice of this exercise.
6. The very important feature of Shirshasana is that it provides systematic flow of blood to brain and nervous system of the body. Hence it controls the mind and body system. Hence this asana is called as "King of asanas." Still many of them fear that performing this exercise causes heart problems and few others fear that this exercise creates problems in the nervous system. All these interpretations are totally wrong. No doubt, initially one may find it difficult to perform this exercise. But with constant practice one can attain perfection and also get the benefit of this yogic practice.

85. CHAKRASANA: (Wheel Posture)

'Chakra' refers to 'Wheel', and in this yogic practice, body should bend and resemble a wheel. This exercise can be done either in standing position or in lying position.

Technique

1. Perform Tadasana.
2. Place the legs apart, about one-foot.
3. Raise the hands above the head. The hands should be straight.
4. Inhale slowly and then bend the body backwards.
5. Slowly bend the body and then place the palm on the ground just behind the ankles.
6. The hands and legs should be erect and firm.
7. Hold in this position for a few seconds with normal breathing. Come back to the normal position and relax.

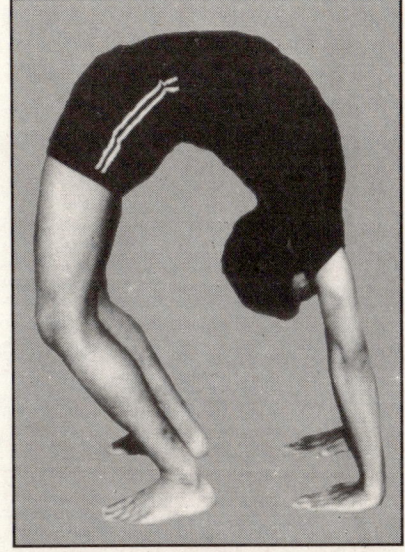
Fig. 85.0

Therapeutic Advantages

1. This exercise is very good for those who are suffering from back pain. In this exercise the entire back position is exercised very well so it is very useful to sportsmen.
2. This exercise helps to correct the disorders of the kidney.
3. Cures the disorders of the neck, shoulder and the spine. It helps to make the spinal column more flexible.
4. It helps to cure throat problems, tonsils and chronic headache.
5. Improves vision power and corrects eye disorders.

86. PURNA CHAKRASANA

Technique

1. Perform Chakrasana (refer Fig. 85.0).
2. Exhale slowly and move the palms so that the palm is near the heels. The crown of the head should be near the hips.
3. The legs and the hands should be firm and stretched well (refer Fig 86.0).
4. Hold in this position for about 8 to 10 seconds with even breathing.

Therapeutic Advantages

Similar to Chakrasana.

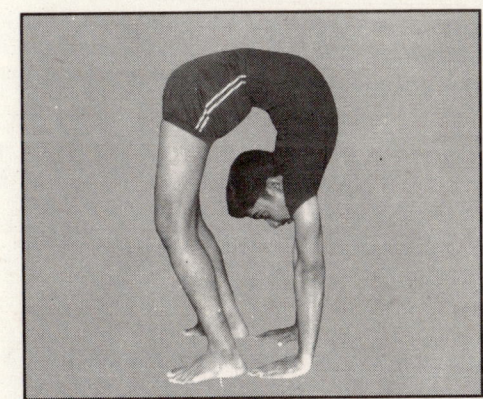
Fig. 86.0

87. VIPARITHA CHAKRASANA

This is the final and advanced posture of Chakrasana. Those who are accustomed to Purna Chakrasana will perform this exercise easily.

Technique

1. After performing Purna Chakrasana slowly slide the legs so that they are straight and firm. The crown of the head should touch the hips (refer Fig. 87.0).
2. Stay in this position for about 8 to 10 seconds and then slowly come back to the first stage of Chakrasana. After that, go back to the normal position and relax.

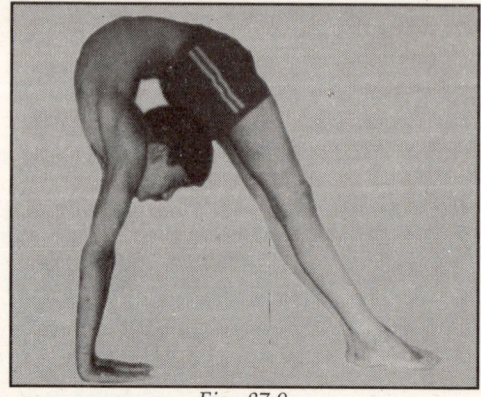
Fig. 87.0

Therapeutic Advantages

1. The advanced posture of Chakrasana helps to provide good body shape.
2. This helps to strengthen the back and eliminates back pain. Helps removal of fat in the hip's region.
3. It provides enough strength to the shoulders, thighs and legs. Hence it is recommended for sportsmen and athletes.

88. SAVITHRASANA

This is one of the most important exercises, which provides balance to the body system and also enhances concentration and thinking power.

Technique

1. Perform Chakrasana (refer Fig. 85.0).
2. Slowly move the palms towards the heels. Simultaneously move the head in between both the legs. Place the forearms on the floor. Lift the head and concentrate on a particular object (refer Fig. 88.0).
3. Come back to Chakrasana and then back to the normal position and relax.

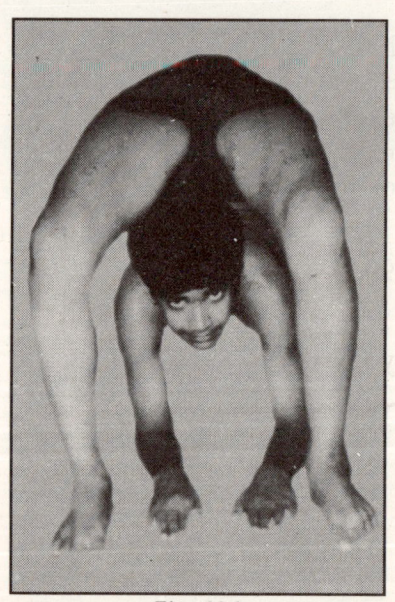
Fig. 88.0

Therapeutic Advantages

1. This exercise gives good nourishment to the legs, knees, back, shoulders and elbows.
2. The entire body is exercised so it provides good body balance and fitness.
3. This helps to enrich flexibility and elasticity to entire body system.
4. This helps to enrich the KUNDALINI POWER and hence it increases the strength and stamina of the body.

89. CHAKRABHANDASANA

Technique

1. Perform Chakrasana (refer Fig. 85.0).
2. Slowly move the hands so that the legs are locked with the hands just above the feet.
3. Raise the head above (refer Fig. 89.0) so that the entire body is stretched well.
4. Stay for a few seconds in this posture with even breathing and then come back to normal position.

Therapeutic Advantages

Chakrasana & Chakrabhandasana have many advantages regarding various disorders of human body system. This exercise helps to eliminate the illness in rectum, kidney, neck and spinal system of the body.

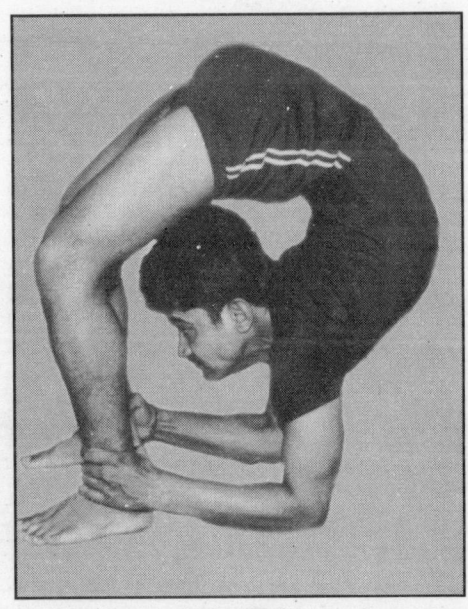

Fig. 89.0

90. GHANDABERUNDASANA

This yogic posture resembles the species of bird. This is one of the difficult yogic exercises, which has several uses.

Technique

1. Perform Chakrabhandasana.
2. Slowly insert the head in between the legs. The heels should touch the shoulder (refer Fig. 90.0).
3. Place the arm straight towards sideways like wings of the bird (refer Fig. 90.1).

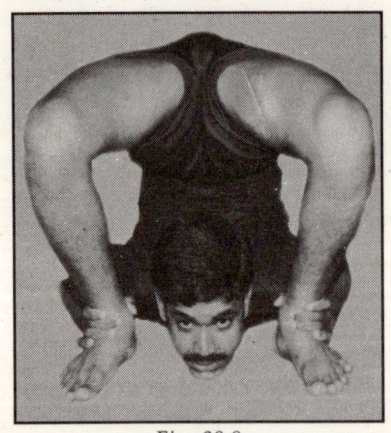
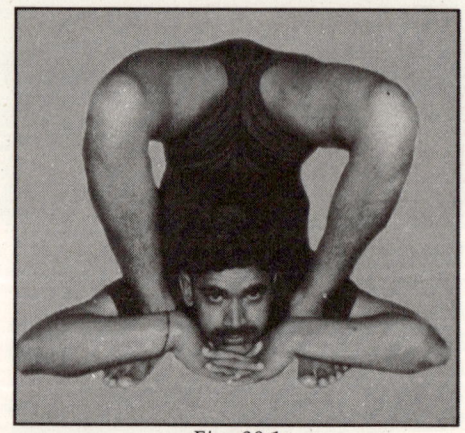

Fig. 90.0   Fig. 90.1

4. Hold in this position for few seconds with normal breathing.
5. Release the interlock and then slowly take back the head from in between the legs. Resume back to Chakrabhandasana. Come back to the normal position and relax.

Therapeutic Advantages

1. The problems in the area of spinal and abdominal organs are cured.
2. This exercise helps to increase vitality.
3. The disorder in the region of pelvic, abdominal region are cured.
4. Practising this exercise helps to increase the KUNDALINI POWER (cosmic energy in the body).

91. TRIANGYA MUKOTHANASANA

'Triang' means 'oblique', 'mukha' denotes the face. Uttana is intense stretch. In this exercise there is an intense stretch of arms, legs and the trunk.

Technique

1. Perform Chakrasana (refer Fig. 85.0).
2. Exhale slowly, stretch the trunk as much as possible in order to bring the hands and catch the shins just above the ankles.
3. Move the head slowly so as to make an effort to take them near the hips (refer Fig. 91.0).
4. Hold in this position for a few seconds. Come back to Chakrasana and relax.

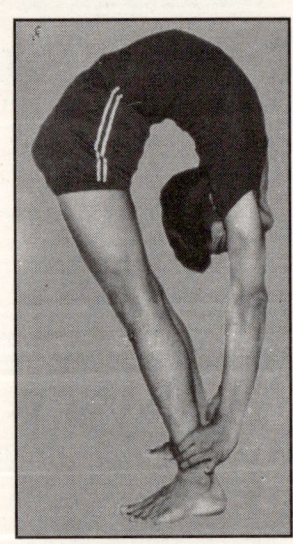

Fig. 91.0

Therapeutic Advantages

1. This exercise helps to strengthen the legs, the thighs and the spine. Hence this exercise is helpful to athletes and sportsmen.
2. Helps to cure joint pain, stiff neck and back pain.
3. Abdominal disorder and disorders in the pelvic region will be effectively cured.

92. PINCHA MAYURASANA: (Half Arm Balance Posture)

Technique

1. Stand firmly on the ground and bend forward. Place the palms on the floor.
2. Exhale slowly, swing the legs up so that the entire body balance is on elbows (refer Fig. 92.0).
3. Hold in this posture for a few seconds, and then slowly come back to the normal position.

Therapeutic Advantages

1. This asana provides enough strength to the shoulders, elbows and to the back.
2. In this exercise abdominal and spinal muscles are stretched, the diseases in those areas are cured.

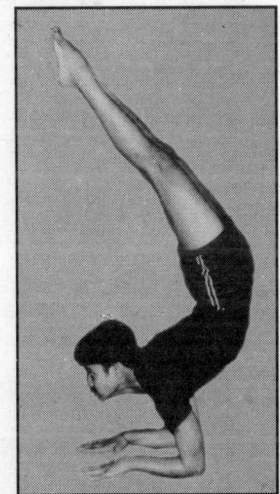

Fig. 92.0

93. ADHOMUKA VRIKSHASANA: (Full Arm Balance Posture)

Technique

1. Stand on the ground, bend forward and place the palm on

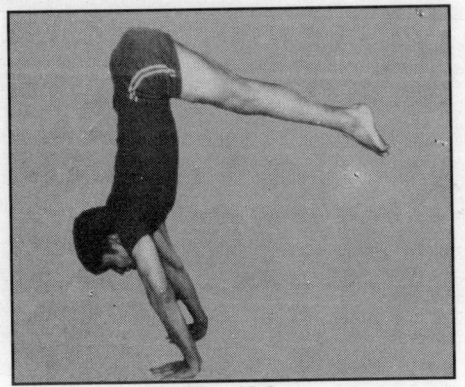

Fig. 93.0

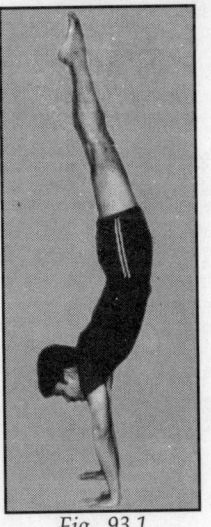

Fig. 93.1

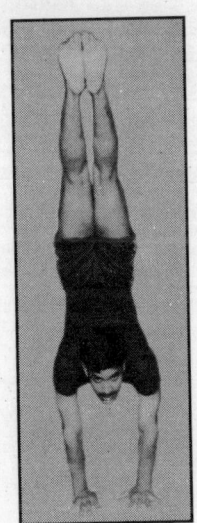

Fig. 93.2

the floor. Raise the legs so that they are horizontal to the ground (refer Fig. 93.0).
2. Exhale slowly and then stretch the legs upward. The entire body balance is on the hands (refer Fig. 93.1 & 93.2).

Caution: This is a difficult exercise, one can experience difficulty in performing this exercise in the initial stages. So it is advisable to practise this exercise with the support of the wall. Once the practice is continued then one can easily practise without any support.

Therapeutic Advantages

Most of the uses are similar to Vrischikasana.

94. VRISCHIKASANA I: (Scorpion Posture)

Technique

1. Perform Pincha Mayurasana (refer Fig. 94.0).
2. Slowly move the legs towards the back so that the feet are placed on the crown of the head.
3. Stay in this position for about 8 to 10 seconds with normal breathing.
4. Resume back the Pincha Mayurasana, then to a normal position.

Therapeutic Advantages

These are given in Vrischikasana II.

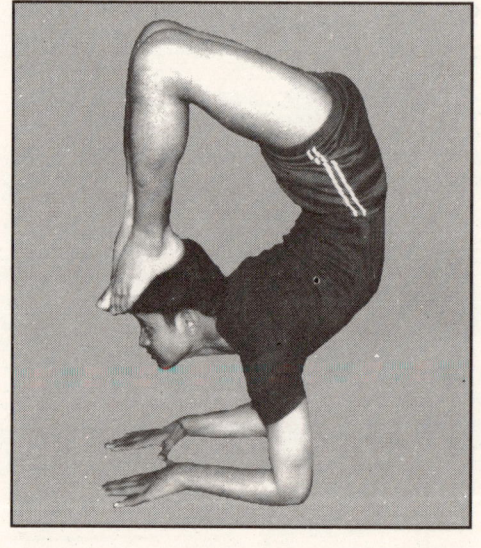

Fig. 94.0

95. VRISCHIKASANA II: (Scorpion Posture)

This is an advanced posture of Vrischikasana.

Technique

1. Perform Adhomuka Vrikshasana. After getting the balance exhale slowly and bend the knees so that the feet rest on the crown of the head (refer Fig. 95.0).
2. Hold in this position for a few seconds, slowly come back to the normal position.

Therapeutic Advantages

1. An effective exercise to cure all spinal problems and abdominal diseases.
2. In Hatha yoga, this exercise is very significant in respect of psychological function of human body. Practising this exercise reduces emotional stress, hatred and depression. It provides concentration, mental peace and tones up the nervous system of the body.
3. The legs, knees and back are stretched in these exercises, the ailments in these areas are cured effectively.

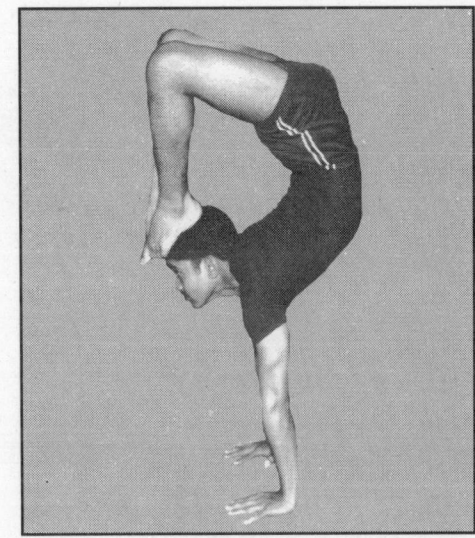

Fig. 95.0

96. PAVANAMUKTHASANA

Technique

1. Lie down on the floor with the face upward. Bend both the knees and wrap the hands around the legs as shown in the posture.
2. Ensure that the hands are locked with the support of fingers.
3. Exhale slowly, raise the head forward till the forehead is in between the knees. The thighs should be pressed against the stomach (refer Fig. 96.1).
4. Inhale deeply and gradually lower the head and relax.
5. Exhale, bring the forehead near the knees. Repeat the process for about 10 times (refer Fig. 96.1).
6. This exercise is performed on each side, wherein each thigh presses against the stomach in Ekapada Pavanamukthasana (refer Fig. 96.0). Those who find it difficult to perform Dwipada Pavanamukthasana, can start with Ekpada Pavanamukthasna (refer Fig. 96.0) and with practice it is easier to perform Dwipada

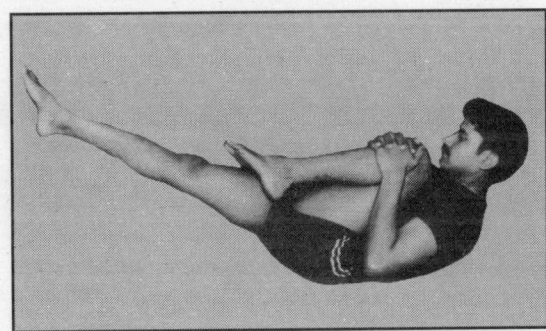

Fig. 96.0 : Ekapada Pavanamukthasana

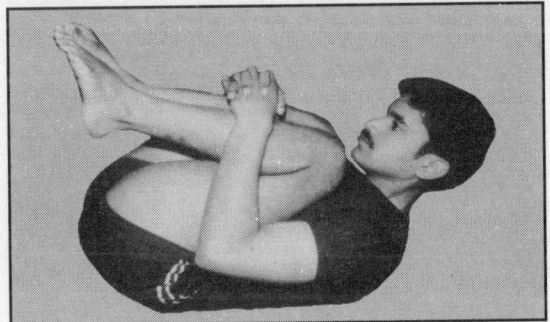

Fig. 96.1 : Dwipada Pavanamukthasana

Pavanamukthasana. Since both the thighs together press against the abdomen, it is called as Dwipada Pavanamukthasana.

Therapeutic Advantages

1. The therapeutic advantages of Ekapada Pavanamukthasana and Dwipada Pavanamukthasana are more or less same.
2. This is an effective exercise to cure constipation and digestive disorders. It cures indigestion and promotes digestive function.
3. In this exercise abdominal region is exercised very well and all the abdominal diseases are cured.
4. It cures gastric trouble and also those suffering from piles get relief.

97. KARNA PEEDASANA: (Ear Posture)

'Karna' refers to the ear and 'pida' means pain or discomfort. The name itself suggests that this is an effective exercise to eliminate all the problems connected with ear.

Technique

1. Start with Sarvangasana (as Fig. 56.0).
2. Bend towards the back on the head and toes should touch the ground. Press the right thigh against right ear and left thigh against left ear. The knees should touch the ground and chin should touch the neck (refer Fig. 97.0).

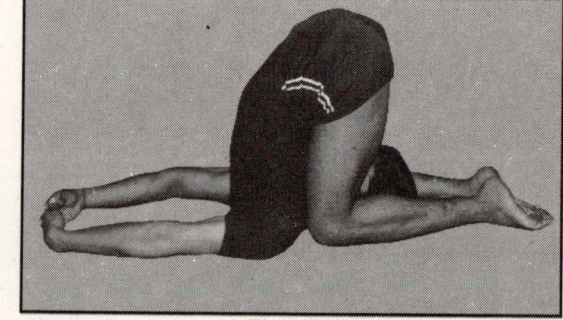

Fig. 97.0

3. Hold about 30 to 40 seconds with normal breathing. Stretch the hands above the head and keep them straight.

Therapeutic Advantages

1. As the name itself suggests, all the ear problems are cured. There will be a definite cure for temporary deafness.
2. The pain in the region of knees, shoulder, and thighs are cured.
3. Cures indigestion and reduces fat in the region of hips.

98. KOUNDINYASANA

Koundinya was a great sage belonging to Vasista family. This yogic exercise is dedicated to sage Koundinya.

Technique

1. Sit on the ground and stretch the legs forward.
2. Exhale slowly, turn the trunk towards the right and place the palms on the ground.
3. Pressing the palms firmly lift the head and also raise the trunk slowly. Ensure that legs are parallel to the floor. The entire body balance rests on the palms.
4. Hold in this position for about 10 to 20 seconds with normal breathing.
5. Repeat the process on the other side also.
6. Slowly lower the legs so as to come back to the normal position.

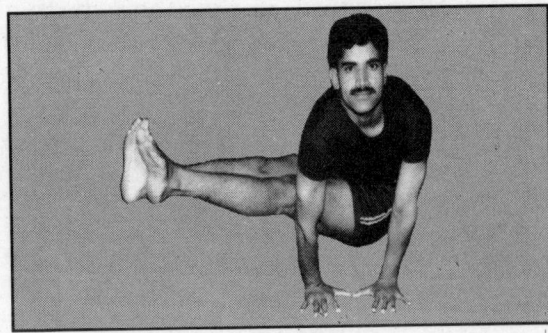
Fig. 98.0

Therapeutic Advantages

1. It gives nourishment to leg muscles, shoulder and hands.
2. Abdominal disorders are cured effectively.
3. Joint pain and arthritis are cured very well.

99. SHIRSHA PADASANA

'Shirsha' means 'head' and 'pada' means 'foot'. In this exercise the foot is to be placed on the crown of the head. Hence it is termed as Shirsha Padasana. Though it resembles Dhanurasana, it has distinct features and advantages.

Technique

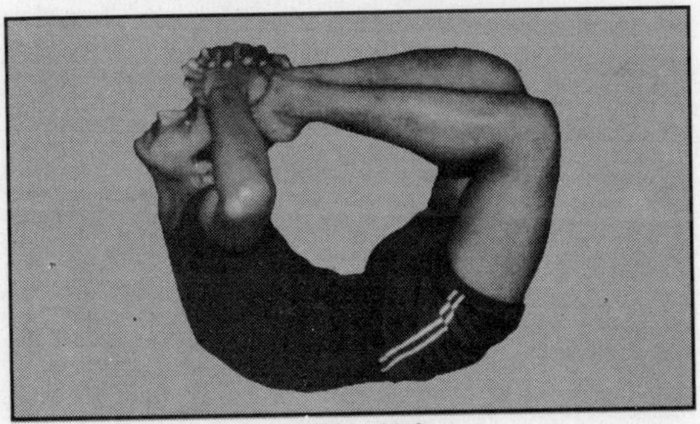

1. Perform Padangusta Dhanurasana (refer Fig. 80.0).
2. Exhale, slowly bend the legs near the knees and place the feet on the crown of the head. The legs should be horizontal to the ground.
3. Place the hands on the foot and make a lock with the help of fingers.
4. Stretch the neck to the maximum extent. There should be perfect arch on the back (refer Fig. 99.0).
5. Hold in this position for 10 to 15 seconds with normal breathing.
6. Slowly release the interlock of the hand and also release the legs and relax.

Fig. 99.0

Therapeutic Advantages

1. This asana helps to strengthen the back, the neck, the shoulder, the thighs and the foot.
2. This exercise is recommended for the disorders of the urinary system.
3. This asana helps to prevent accumulation of fat in the region of stomach and hips.
4. It helps to cure congested liver, spleen and other related problem.

100. SHAVASANA: (Corpse Pose—Complete Relaxation Posture)

In Sanskrit 'Shava' means a 'Dead body'. Here in this exercise one has to lie down like a dead body in order to get complete relaxation. The purpose of performing various yogic exercises is for the intention to obtain good health, mental happiness and also to get relaxation. Shavasana is performed after completion of all the yogic exercises. During the present busy life no one is able to experience complete relaxation, even though many comforts are available to us. But only the physical comforts alone cannot provide complete relaxation. Complete relaxation can be experienced only when both physical and mental relaxations are attained. In medical sciences it is generally believed that when there is a mental relaxation most of the dreadful diseases are cured without any medicines. Shavasana which is a very important yogic practice provides the complete method of total relaxation.

The process and method of Shavasana appears to be simple but it is not so easy to practise. Mere sleeping does not constitute Shavasana. The exact systematic process of Shavasana is explained below.

Technique

1. Lie flat on the floor with the face upward. The whole body must be loose, at ease, and straight (refer Fig. 100).
2. Close the eyes and breathe slowly and evenly.
3. Ensure that all the parts of the body, that is, from head to toe are relaxed. The mind should be calm and vacant. The unnecessary thinking or worldly interest should be completely avoided.
4. Start consciously relaxing each part of the body starting from head to toes and experience the total relaxation of each and every part of the body.
5. It is very essential that there should not be any outside disturbance while

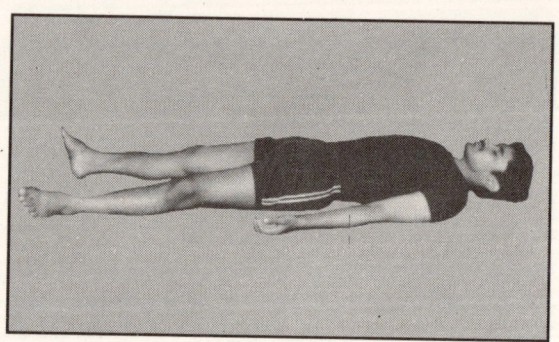

Fig. 100

doing any yogic exercise, particularly Shavasana.
6. Lie in this posture for about 10-15 minutes or more till one finds complete relaxation of the entire body.

Therapeutic Advantages

1. Provides total and complete relaxation to body and mind which helps to cure several health problems, particularly nervous disorders, blood pressure, insomnia, relief from strain and fatigue, gastric trouble.
2. Provides energy and freshness to the body and mind.
3. Rhythmic breathing helps to tone up the respiratory system.

5

Eye Care—Exercises

The eye is an important sensory organ which is most essential to everyone. It is the duty of everyone to protect his eyes and nourish them in order to maintain visual power of the eyes. Nowadays most of them are facing visual troubles even at the childhood stage.

There are many reasons for visual troubles. The important factors for visual problem, include:

1. Hereditary Reasons: Visual defects, which are due to hereditary reasons, and in this case the visual defects may appear in the early stage.

2. Eye Strain: The reasons under this head are plenty. Usage of eyes improperly, working in a polluted atmosphere, viewing television for long durations and working on computers for longer periods etc. are some of the reasons which cause visual defects. Unfortunately, most of the people are under the impression that using glasses or spectacles is the only remedy available to rectify the visual defects. No doubt, using glasses help to give good vision, but it cannot help to eliminate the visual problems.

In **Yoga Shastra** we come across references about sensory organs, more particularly about visual power. According to **Yoga Shastra** there are two kinds of eyes, namely, the external and the internal. The structure of that we see from outside is the external eye and the invisible force that gives command to the eyes from the mind is referred as inner eye. In yogic science the visual defects can be corrected by enriching the sensory perception through variety of yogic exercises.

Yogic Exercise for Better Eyesight

1. Palming: This is the simple and the initial stage of eye exercise. When the eyes are strained or exhausted, they require relaxation. In such cases, closing the eyes by placing the palms on both the eyes for two to three minutes, helps to relax our eyes. While being palmed, the eyes should be closed first, and then place the palm covering the eyes without putting any pressure around the eyes. Ensure that the outside light does not reach the eyes.

2. Central Fixation: Normally when we see a thing, our eyes are focussed only on that part of the object. Place the 'OM' chart in a convenient place where sufficient natural light is available.

Stand in front of the chart by keeping normal distance. Start shifting the sight on the angular lines of the OM chart. Focus each line of the chart perfectly while shifting, move the head and sight together. Blink the eyes evenly and ensure that the eyes are not strained while performing central fixation.

3. Sun Treatment: Our eyes are so sensitive, it cannot withstand bright light or total darkness. In yogic science we know that Sun provides energy to the human body. No doubt Sun gives energy to our eyes also. This exercise should be done during early in the morning, that is, at the time of sunrise.
  i. Stand towards the direction of sun.
  ii. Close the eyes and lift the head slowly towards the direction of the sun.
  iii. Slowly start shifting the head towards sideways and also forward and backward directions. Swinging should be done for about two to three minutes. After completion of swinging, start blinking fast for about a minute. Take complete relaxation for about one minute.

4. Lamp/Candle Exercises (Thrataka)
  i. Place lighting candle/lamp on a table.
  ii. Sit in front of the candle by maintaining a distance of about 5 to 6 feet.
  iii. Start exercise by closing the eyelids. Open the eyes slowly and concentrate on the outer surface of the lamp flame for about a minute.
  iv. Close the eyes and perform palming. After that relax the eyes for about a minute.
  v. Slowly open the eyelids, focussing central part of the candle flame for about a minute. While focussing towards the flames of the lamp, blinking of eyes should not be done. After performing this exercise give rest to the eyes. Perform this exercise for about 5 to 6 times.

5. Swinging
  i. Stand in front of a window having vertical iron bars.
  ii. Stand with feet apart and start sway gently from one side to the other.

iii. While swinging one should look beyond and through the bars. While doing so blink at each end.
iv. Perform this exercise for about 3 to 5 minutes.
v. Moving of eyes upward and downward, moving towards right corner upward and left corner downward and circular movements of the eyes (clockwise and anti-clockwise) will help to increase the sharpness of the eyes. Perform this upward and downward as well as circular movement of the eyes for about 3 to 5 minutes. After performing this exercise relax the eyes for about a minute.

6. Rotation of Head: Both clockwise and anti-clockwise rotation will help to improve the eyesight. First start the rotation of head in a clockwise direction for about a minute and then relax the eyes by palming. After relaxation start rotating the head in anti-clockwise direction.

7. Eye Wash: Washing the eyes is very important to maintain health of the eyes. Take pure water in a eye wash cup. Bend the head and dip the eyes in the water. Blink gently in the water. Wash the eyes for about one to two minutes.

8. Yogic Exercises for Better Eyesight:
   i. Surya Namaskar.
   ii. Simhasana(29)
   iii. Mayurasana(33)
   iv. Shirshasana(84)
   v. Sarvangasana(56)
   vi. Paschimothanasana(38)
   vii. Matsyasana(30)
   viii. Ustrasana(43)
   ix. Dhanurasana(79)
   x. Shavasana(100)

9. Pranayama

10. Meditation

6

Pranayama

In Sanskrit 'prana' refers to the cosmic energy, that we also call as 'Breath'. 'Ayama' means to control the prana i.e., to control the breathing. Every living creature has to breathe for existence. Breathing is a continuous process, which provides vital energy to the body. From various studies we come to conclusion that pranayama refers to controlling of the breath.

The concept of pranayama, which is derived from "Pranasya ayamah pranayama" i.e., command or mastery over prana, is pranayama. One who controls his own breath is nothing but a perfect stage of pranayama. How to control prana, i.e., the breath, is the essence of pranayama. From the studies of olden epics and Vedas it was known that the prana is the integral part of all human existence and also to attain moksha. In **Atharva Veda 18.2.56** it is rightly said:

> "O man, I yoke thy soul that goes to the next
> World through breath, with two carriers,
> The Prana and Apana.
> Through this control through yoga,
> Seek shelter under God common with him!

Every living creature knowingly or unknowingly requires breathing without any break. We have read in several books and also concluded from various scientific studies that oxygen is required for breathing, more than that for our existence. But we do not know how to breathe and the concept of breathing and the advantages of systematic breathing. In pranayama one does not only learn the art of breathing but also gains command over one's own Prana. Hence pranayama is considered as an important concept in yoga and meditation.

> "The pure soul, cleaned through the control of
> Breath and meditation soon attains salvation
> And becomes one with God through yogic Samadhi."
> [Atharva. 6.51.1]

From the above Vedic verse we came to know that the Soul can be cleaned and attain salvation through control of breath. For all the living creatures the Prana is the vital force of existence, without which there will be an end of life.

Regarding the process of breathing and respiration there are scores of research studies available all over the world. Even the advanced medical research agrees that breathing is an art, a systematic breathing alone controls entire human body system. From various studies we come to know that the normal rate of respiration is about 16 to 20 cycles per minute and during sleeping the rate comes down to 10 to 12 cycle per minute and in deep meditation the rate comes down to 4 to 6 cycle per minute. That is, during the stage of meditation or during utmost concentration of mind one can control his own breath, which is nothing but a stage of control over mind and body. From this we can come to conclusion that there is a relationship between pranayama and meditation.

The pranayama is the main part of the yogic science and many researches have already been done in this area. Here an attempt has been made to explain in short, the basic values and advantages of pranayama.

FEATURES OF PRANAYAMA

There are four important features of pranayama which give us the techniques of breath regulation.

1. Slowing of Breath: In pranayama control of breath is a very important concept. In the olden Puranas it was said that yogic breathing is the technique which brings to control all that is connected with the prana. Breathing inward is known as 'Puraka', breathing outward is called as 'Rechaka'. Retaining or holding the breath in the lungs is 'Kumbaka'. When one who holds his breath beyond one's capacity, rechaka becomes fast and uncontrolled. Here the important point is that, one has to slow down the rate of respiration in order to bring down the metabolic rate of the body. This can be done by holding kumbaka. The breathing rate is directly proportional to the metabolic process of human body. The reduction in metabolic rate will serve as a measure of rest. Thus slowing down the breath gives deep rest to the body and mind.

2. Consciousness of Breathing: This important concept provides to know the awareness of breathing. From the studies of Hatha yoga we came to know that holding of breath i.e. Kumbaka will help to build the awareness.

In Vasista Pranayama, holding of breath for certain duration is not mandatory. Alternatively the breath has to be slowed down continuously both during inhalation and exhalation, keeping in mind about relaxation. Here in Vasista Pranayama holding the breath with certain amount of effort is not the requirement. But slowing down the breath in the continuous process of respiration without any effort is safe.

3. Balancing the Breath: The breathing process will be done through the two nostrils. There has been a debate whether the breathing through both the nostrils is same or not. From the yogic studies we came to know that inhaling from the right nostril produces heat in the body whereas inhaling from the left nostril produces cold. Whatever may be the consequences, the nadishudhi in Pranayama deals with the cleaning of two nadis that is *ida* and *Pingala* in order to bring balance of breath.

4. Breath Meditation: Earlier we came to know the art of holding of the breath, creation of breath awareness and balancing the breath. We know that breathing is for our existence. Systematic breathing controls entire function of the human body. From meditation one can attempt to control his mind. When the mind is controlled our breathing will be controlled. When our mind is agitated or disturbed then our breathing will be fast and unequal. The purpose of Pranayama is to control and regulate the breathing to attain the mind control. Controlling the mind on the contrary controls the breathing system.

PRACTICE OF PRANAYAMA

The first and important point before practising pranayama—one has to get the complete knowledge about the process, methods, functions and requirements of Pranayama from any yoga practitioner. Practice of Pranayama under the guidance of expert yoga professional is the basic ingredient. Without such guidance and support, practising Pranayama will not provide any benefit or advantage, because in Pranayama the entire concept is on regulation of breathing which has to be taught by some one who is an expert in Pranayama.

Secondly, the place chosen to perform Pranayama must be very clean, peaceful, ventilated and also free from dust and moisture.

Thirdly, performing Pranayama in the early morning, preferably before sunrise is the ideal time. Those who find it difficult to perform Pranayama in the morning, can practise in the evening also.

Fourthly, Pranayama can be done either in Padmasana, Vajrasana, Siddhasana or in Sukhasana posture. Out of these the convenient posture has to be opted first. While practising pranayama eyes must be closed and breathing should be normal. Ensure the entire body is relaxed and at peace.

Fifthly, the most important factor while performing pranayama is to maintain concentration and mental peace. Here the practitioner has to control the breathing system in order to harness benefits of Pranayama.

Sixthly, Pranayama can be performed after three to four hours gap after taking the food. Better to avoid "Shitakari" and "Sitali" Pranayama, during winter season and "Surya Bhedhana" Pranayama during summer.

ADVANTAGES OF PRANAYAMA

In Pranayama, the systematic system of breathing is gained. The systematic breathing function gives complete physical and mental relaxation to the human body.

The healthy and systematic breathing tones up the entire respiratory function of the body, and all the disorders in respiratory function are completely eliminated.

Pranayama is most effective for digestion and other digestive disorders. In the process of Pranayama the digestive organs, more particularly diaphragm and abdominal muscles are toned up which helps to cure disorders in stomach, pancreas, liver and kidney.

Regular and constant practice of Pranayama helps to ensure proper distribution of blood to all the nerves and glands evenly, hence all the nervous disorders will be effectively cured. The Brain, Spinal column and the entire nervous system of the body are toned up and they will function properly.

The systematic yogic breathing in Pranayama helps to nourish the body and mind. In the process of Pranayama more and more oxygen flows into the body, which helps to relieve the muscle pain, fatigue and other disorders.

There are several other advantages of Pranayama which have been explained under various methods.

THE NADIS, CHAKRAS AND BANDHAS

Every Pranayama practitioner must have knowledge of nadis, chakras and bandhas which is necessary for perfect practice of Pranayama.

Bandhas: Bandha means bondage or joining together. In Bandhas wherein certain parts of the body are controlled, while performing Pranayama in order to check the dissipation of human energy, it is required to apply Bandhas in order to get the maximum benefits of Pranayama. There are three types of Bandhas:
- Uddiyana Bandha
- Jalandhara Bandha
- Mula Bandha

Uddiyana Bandha: In Sanskrit Uddiyana refers to flying up. That is, here in this Bandha lift the diaphragm, thorax highup and pull the abdominal organ against the back towards the spine. This process involves contraction of pelvis (lower abdomen).

Jalandhara Bandha: Jala means a net or a web. In Jalandhara Bandha the head should be lower down towards front and chin should rest on the chest in the notch between the collarbones and at the top of the breastbone.

Mula Bandha: In Sanskrit Mula means the origin or a root. Mula Bandha is the region between the anus and scrotum. Here the technique involves the contraction of anus.

Nadis: The human body consists of countless nadis and all such nadis have their own functions and significance. Among the countless nadis the most important nadis are:

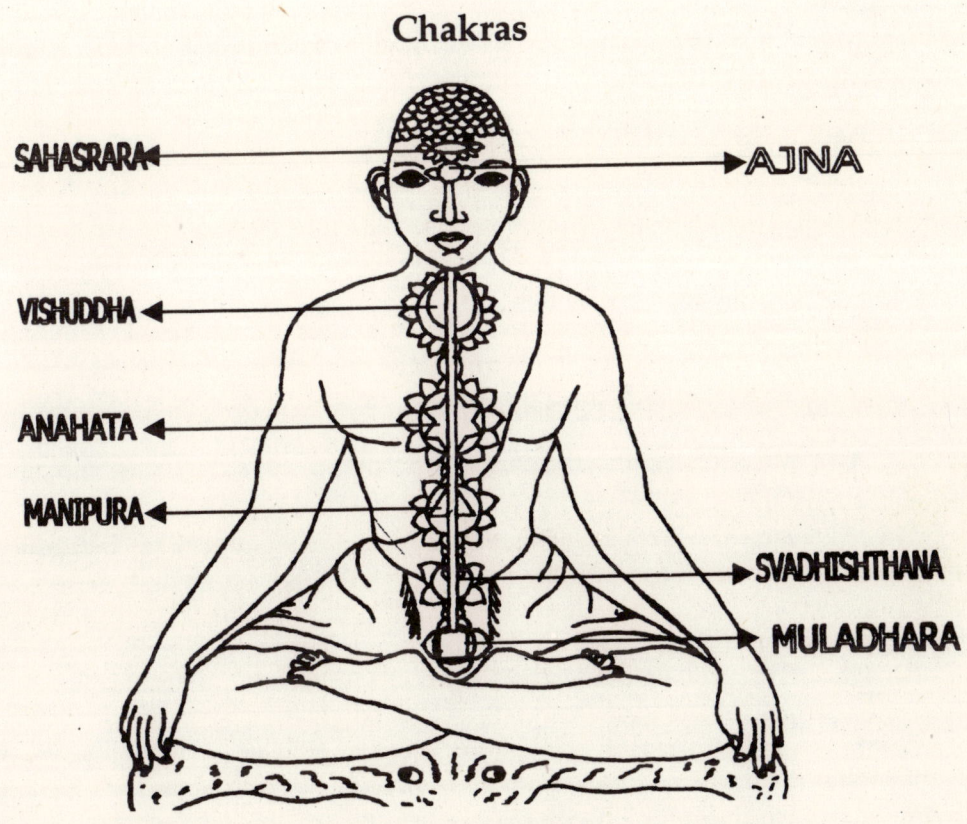

THE YOGA CHAKRAS

The Ida: Situated at the left side of the spinal column.
Pingala: Situated at the right side of spinal column.
Sushumna: Situated in the middle of the spinal column.

In the epics as well as in several yogic studies, Pingala is termed as Nadi of the Sun, Ida is the Nadi of the Moon and Sushumna is the Nadi of the Fire. The junctions of Ida, Pingala and Sushumna are called Chakras.

In meditation as well as in yogic science, Chakras are very significant. Great yogies and sages practiced meditation by concentrating on the chakras to attain Moksha and realisation of God. There are seven important chakras and each of the chakras symbolizes the particular parts of the human body.

Muladhara: Situated at the base of the spine, that is, in the pelvic region.
Swadhisthaya: Situated between the navel and the genital organs.
Manipuraka: Situated in the area of navel.
Anantha: Situated in the heart region.
Vishuddha: Situated in the throat, that is, in the pharyngeal region.
Ajna: Situated in between the eyebrows.
Sahasrara: Situated on the top of the head, that is, in the cerebral cavity.

IMPORTANT METHODS AND CONCEPTS OF PRANAYAMA

In Pranayama there are several methods and procedures out of which few of them are explained to provide complete knowledge of Pranayama.

PURAKA, RECHAKA AND KUMBAKA: [Inhalation, exhalation and retention of breath]

Inhalation and exhalation, though is a continuous process of breathing for one's existence, in Pranayama these aspects have been given a special significance. Breathing is a systematic process. In Pranayama, it gives adequate knowledge about systematic inhalation and exhalation and also how to hold the breath in order to get human energy development and attain concentration.

The deep inhalation process which is generally termed in **Brihadyagiyanyavalkya Smrithi** as "Sucking the air from the environment with the aid of nose and making it fill all the Nadis in the body is the puraka variety of control of breath."

Rechaka refers to "An exhalation of breath where the air is thrown to the atmosphere from the human body."

Puraka and Rechaka is a continuous process, that is, taking breath inside and throwing the air from the body, which controls entire functions of the body. After inhalation and exhalation process, the next advanced concept of Pranayama is Kumbaka. Here in between the inhalation and exhalation process, the control of breath is very important. It is not easy to hold the breath while the inhalation and exhalation process is going on. But in yogic science it rightly said that holding of breath helps to provide benefit to the human body. But the question is how much the breath should be held? And for how many seconds it should be held? These are the significant concepts in Kumbaka system. The control of breath, which is the main essence of Pranayama, provides information regarding art of breathing technique and holding of breath which is very beneficial to each and every one.

Earlier we have discussed several concepts of Pranayama, which ensures good health to everyone. But quite often the question arises in our mind regarding the practice of Pranayama. Firstly and more importantly the Pranayama should be done exclusively under the supervision of Pranayama expert in order to attain full benefits of Pranayama. Failing which the very purpose of performing Pranayama will be defeated. More than that without such guidance performing Pranayama may not yield any benefit, but even adversely affect the physical functions of the body. Here an attempt is made to explain the basic methods of Pranayama.

1. ANULOMA-VILOMA PRANAYAMA

Sit in any convenient yogic posture. Place the hands on the knees, the body should be straight.

Technique

1. Exhale slowly and completely through both the nostrils.
2. Immediately thereafter start inhaling by abdominal breathing.
3. While breathing ensure not to make any noise or strain.
4. Once the inhalation is completed, the air should not be retained in the lungs but immediately exhalation should be continued.

Make sure the breathing is deep and uniform. The alternate exhalation and inhalation is the simplest type of Pranayama.

Therapeutic Advantages

1. It cleans the respiratory system.
2. Tones up the nervous system of the body.
3. It helps to cure serious and recurring headache.

2. UJJAYI PRANAYAMA (Energy Renewing Pranayama)

Technique

1. Sit in any of the convenient yogic posture viz, Padmasana or Siddhasana or Vajrasana.
2. The air in the lungs should be exhaled through both the nostrils and then inhaled slowly through both the nostrils. The inhalation will be for 3-4 seconds. Inhaling of air should be done by abdominal breathing. Once inhalation is completed, perform Mula Bandha, the anus should be contracted, simultaneously the breath should be held in the lungs with Jalandhara Bandha by pressing the chin against the chest. Now retain the air in Kumbaka for a period of 10 to 15 seconds.
3. Release the bandhas and start exhalation slowly by performing 'uddiyana bandha'. The exhalation can be done for the period of 8 to 10 seconds. The exhalation should be done through the left nostril while right nostril will

be closed by right thumb. Please note that in ujjayi Pranayama inhalation is always from both nostrils where as the exhalation is only through the left nostril.

Therapeutic Advantages

1. Ujjayi Pranayama is more effective to control entire nervous system.
2. Those who suffer from blood pressure, the regular and systematic practice of Pranayama will cure the blood pressure and the other disorders.
3. The chronic asthma, cough and other respiratory disorders will get cured.

3. SURYA BHEDHANA PRANAYAMA
(Breathing that Activates the Nervous System)

'Surya' refers to the 'sun' and 'Bhedhana', means to 'open'. In this Pranayama the breathing process involves inhalation through left nostrils.

Technique

Sit in Vajrasana or in any convenient yogic posture. In this Pranayama exhalation is the first process, that is, one has to exhale completely. Close the left nostril with the help of left-hand thumb and start inhaling through right nostril. After inhaling is completed, immediately perform mula bandha and jalandhara bhanda. While doing so the right nostril should be closed with the help of middle finger of the left hand. By doing so the breath can be kept under retention and preferably retain the breath for about 15 to 20 seconds. Slowly unlock the bandha. With the help of right nostril, start exhalation for about 8 seconds. This completes one cycle of breathing under surya-bhedhana Pranayama. Repeat this breathing cycle for about 10 times.

Therapeutic Advantages

1. In this Pranayama, the advantage is that the entire body temperature is kept under control, so that it helps the nervous system and digestive system of the body.
2. The respiratory disorders, recurring cold, partial headache and throat pain get cured.

4. CHANDRA BHEDHANA PRANAYAMA

'Chandra' means the 'moon', 'Bhedhana' refers 'to open'. In this Pranayama the excess body heat is removed.

Technique

1. Sit in Vajrasana or in any convenient yogic posture.
2. Close the right nostril and start inhaling through the left nostril for about 4 to 5 seconds. Perform Kumbaka for 10 to 15 seconds by adopting the Bandhas and closing the left nostril.
3. Slowly start unlocking the Bandhas and then start exhalation through the left nostril for 6 to 8 seconds. It completes one cycle of breathing. Similarly continue the same process for about 5 to 10 times.

Therapeutic Advantages

1. Since the entire excess body heat is removed, the diseases due to body heat like nasal bleeding, burning of eyes etc. will be cured.
2. Loss of hair due to body heat and skin diseases can be cured.
3. Blood pressure, sleeplessness, nervous diseases are also effectively cured.

5. SITALI (Refreshness of Breath)

In this Pranayama the breath will be refreshed and by refreshment of breath the entire body system is refreshed. The breathing should be through the mouth and not through the nose.

Technique

1. Sit in Vajrasana or in any convenient yogic posture.
2. Stretch the tongue and start inhaling slowly so that one can feel the inhalation process. Once the inhalation is completed, close the lips and hold the breath for a few seconds. Slowly start exhalation through both the nostrils. This completes one cycle of breathing. Repeat this process for 6 to 7 times.

Therapeutic Advantages

1. This Pranayama helps refresh the entire body system. All the disorders of liver and spleen are cured. It helps to cure low fever and piles.
2. Since the breathing is through the mouth, the bad odour of the mouth will be cleaned. It also strengthens the vocal chords.

6. SHEETHKARI PRANAYAMA

This Pranayama too eliminates the excess body heat of the human body.

Technique

1. Sit in Vajrasana or in any convenient yogic posture.
2. Exhale completely through both the nostrils.
3. Start inhaling through the mouth with the tip of the tongue pressed against the teeth. Feel the inhaling process and then close the lips. Hold the breath for 3 to 5 seconds.
4. Slowly start exhaling through both the nostrils.
5. Repeat the process for about 8 to 10 times.

Therapeutic Advantages

Similar to Sitali Pranayama.

7. SADHANTHA PRANAYAMA

This Pranayama will eliminate the excess body heat.

Technique

1. Sit in Vajrasana or in any convenient yogic posture.
2. Exhale completely through both the nostrils.
3. Close the upper and lower teeth firmly and start inhalation through the gaps of the teeth. Once the inhalation is completed, hold the breath for about 3 to 5 seconds.
4. Start exhalation slowly through both the nostrils.

Therapeutic Advantages

Similar to Sitali Pranayama.

8. BHAMARI PRANAYAMA

'Bhamari' means the 'Bee'. While breathing it resembles the sound of bee so it is popularly known as Bhamari. In Hatha Yoga Deepika those who practise Bhamari will experience pleasure and happiness. So it is considered as an important yogic Pranayama.

Technique

1. Sit in Vajrasana or in any convenient yogic posture.
2. Close both the ears with the help of big thumb.
3. The body should be straight and relaxed.
4. By making the sound of a bee start inhaling through both the nostrils. Once the inhaling is completed hold the breath for about 3 to 5 seconds.

5. Start exhaling by making the sound of a bee.
6. Repeat this process for about 5 to 8 times.

9. NADISHODHANA PRANAYAMA:
(Cleansing Blood Vessels and Arteries)

In this Pranayama the entire blood vessels and arteries are cleansed and the entire nervous system is toned up. It is the breathing system that regulates the entire body functions. This Pranayama provides the system of breathing to everyone.

Technique

1. Sit in Padmasana or any meditation posture. The body should be straight and relaxed.
2. Exhale completely.
3. Close the right nostril and start inhalation through left nostril and once the inhalation is completed, hold the breath for about 3 to 4 seconds.
4. Release the thumb from right nostril and then close the left nostril. Start exhalation through the right nostril.
5. Once the exhalation is completed, start inhalation through the right nostril by closing the left nostril. Then release the left nostril and start exhaling through left nostril. Continue the process for about 8 to 10 minutes.

Therapeutic Advantages

1. Basically it tones up the blood vessels, veins and arteries so that it helps the body to become immune to all the physical disorders.
2. It activates digestive system and helps to eliminate stomach disorders and disorders of liver and intestine.
3. Helps to cure headache, cold and other respiratory disorders.

7

Meditation

We come across various types of people in the society, and their reactions, responses, behaviour, attitudes, and approaches are different from each other. In our society everyone should anticipate to live together and to share the happiness and agony among each other equally. This will be the main theme of "live and let live". But unfortunately in the present disturbed pattern of living, large scale violence, hatred and egoism and recurring religious conflicts, we are witnessing violence, quarrel, and unrest in every part of the world. This is ultimately creating agitation in the mind and tendency to fight for mean reasons. Man has gone to the level of killing his own parents, brothers or fellow beings without any reason. This is the sad plight of the entire human set up. The reason for the abnormal behaviour of mankind is mainly due to lack of control over mind, lack of thinking power, lack of awareness, lack of philosophical knowledge and lack of unity. These few aspects lead to erosion of human values. Hence, there is a need to develop human mind so that we can develop peace and harmony among all the people of the society. The meditation or Dhyana serves as a powerful weapon to eliminate all such unpleasant things in the society and helps to live peacefully and happily.

The values of meditation that we hear from various religious leaders and organizations claim that meditation provides concentration of mind, health and happiness. Various schools of meditation signify the pattern of meditation in different forms. But whatever may be their principles, methods and procedures, the ultimate objectives of all such meditation are same. If you take the example of Maharshi Mahesh yogi's Transcendental meditation, Rishi Prabhakar's concepts of meditation or thoughts of any school of meditation, the basic concept is to control the mind. When the mind is controlled, then one can restrain from bad thinking, unholy physical pleasure and then it helps to control the soul. When the body and mind are controlled one can attain the state of Nirvikalpa Samadhi, that is the highest stage of meditation (Dhyana). In this stage one can realize the truth and perfection.

All the yogic teachers, practitioners and different schools of meditation express the need for control of mind which is the essence of meditation. But in reality control of mind is a difficult task. Without our knowledge, thoughts and actions come to our mind. A few of such thoughts are good and most other were unwanted. When such thoughts come to our mind, we can suddenly start to execute such thoughts without taking any decision. Because of this reason, nowaday, people are losing their thinking power, which is ultimately resulting in several disturbances in the society. When one loses control over his mind, he will virtually lose control on all the human functions in the society. Lord Shankara rightly said;

"If the mind is in a state of torpor it should be woken up. If it gets dispersed amongst objects, it should be calmed down. If it is latent with the seed of desire, that condition should be recognised. If it is equipped it should be left undisturbed."

It is really difficult to control our desires and to reach the perfect stage of meditation. Simply praying to God or chanting doesn't constitute meditation. Prayer is an ingredient to remember our favourite God, which serves as an aid to control our mind. But one should remember, a true prayer needs a still mind. That is, mind should be fully controlled and it should be in a meditative mind. During the process of meditation the urge and the soul conviction is to control the mind by deviating from the stage of torpor. In our olden epic it was suggested that performing or chanting the sacred God helps to arrest the deviation of mind, that's why the meditation is regarded as a sacred practice which can be attained by systematic control of mind and body.

In **Svetasvthara Upanishad** it is said:

'Na Samdrse tisthati rupamesya
na caksusa pasyati kascanainam;
Hrda manasabhiklrpto
ya etat viduh amrtaste bhavanti'

That is, "His form is not to be seen. No one sees him by the eye. Those who know him by mind as dwelling in the heart become immortal." That is, one who attains concentration of mind always has knowledge of everything and also emerges pure in mind and thought. It is in the stage of perfect meditation and in this stage one can attain samadhi or the supreme. This too is referred in **Bhagvad Gita** as follows.

"Yada bhutaprthagbhavam
Ekasthamanupasyati
Tata eva ca vistaram
Brahma Sampadyate tada."

Whenever a man sees the existence of different beings as rooted in the supreme God he thinks that all beings are projection from him. The moment he attains the supreme, that is the ideal mysticism in meditation, which helps to attain supreme.

All the yoga teachers and schools of yoga emphasize the need for meditation which is the integral part of yoga. In our olden epics as well as in **Yoga Shastra** the references have been found that yoga and meditation serve as a tool for body and mind control. So meditation has occupied an important concept in yogic science. Like control of body, control of mind is very essential. If any one thing is not found, the real essence of yoga itself will be defeated. In the yogic epic we come across two concepts viz, self-restraints [Atma Sangama] and breath control [pranayama]. These two aspects are equally important, i.e. control of body and mind.

In **Bhagvad Gita** lot of references on meditation have been widely discussed. In each and every verse the control of mind, the command over body and mind, and meditation has been widely discussed in the fifth chapter of **Bhagvad Gita**, which is termed as Dhyana yoga, or science of meditation. In Dhyana yoga, in one of the verses it was said;

"Keeping the external contacts with sense objects outside, fixing his sight at the juncture of the eyebrows and making equal the outgoing and incoming breaths passing through the nostrils, the sage whose senses, mind and intellect are controlled. Whose highest control is liberation, from whom desire, fear and anger have gone away and who remains always thus is verily liberated."

This context clarifies the relationship between yoga and meditation. By controlling the breath, concentration and knowledge united together, one can establish control over mind and body. At the outset it seems very difficult to control body and mind easily. But from the studies of our epics, thoughts of our sages, saints and religious leaders, we can understand their efforts to reach the stage of Moksha or liberation from birth and death. Here, our concern is to provide information about how to concentrate the mind. It is no doubt impossible to leave all our desires and interests totally out of our mind. Our idea is to provide systematic and scientific concept to regulate body and mind.

Manu in his Epic says:

"By Pranayamas let him destroy defects [Dosha],
By concentration [Dharana], the sins,
By Dissociation [Prathyhara] sense of attachment,
By meditation [Dhyana], attributes not divine."

He explained the process of cleaning the body and control of mind to acquire knowledge. Meditation involves both physical and mental process. When the body and mind are free from unusual activities, the mind eliminates all the wordly thoughts, which lead to attaining the perfect state of meditation or super sensuous state.

Earlier we have discussed the concept of meditation and its requirement to control our mind. In the present age all are suffering from stress and strain. The school going kids and children loaded with burdensome curriculum, youths facing lot of uncertainty about their future, working professionals overburdened with their work, housewives facing a lot of humiliation and responsibilities on their shoulder, business people facing lot of uncertain and difficult situations. And finally our old aged people are entangled in a lot of psychological and family tension. That is, all classes of people are facing their own problems and tension. They want to be liberated from such anxiety and tension. For this they are seeking the help of yoga and meditation presently available at various yogic institutions. The sad plight that we are witnessing nowadays, is commercialization of yoga and meditation. The progress of science and technology has no doubt provided human advancement in all the areas. In addition to this, such advancement is creating lot of tension and stress among all the sections of the society. The bad plight that we face today is use of scientific equipment and mechanical aid for yoga and meditation, which is spoiling the real and traditional system of yoga and meditation.

In yogic exercise the main concept is to control body in order to gain control over the mind. The basic purpose to perform all yogic exercises is that, one is required to control the mind. Otherwise whatever efforts that can be put, will be wasteful. The quality of yoga, depends on two factors, that is, control of mind and control of body. Without controlling body and mind, no one could get the real benefits of yoga and meditation.

The frequent question that arises in our mind is that, why meditation should be practiced? We have read that control of body and mind is the essence of yoga. We control our body by performing various yogic exercises. Alternatively, to get the benefits of yoga one has to have control over his mind, which ultimately helps to control the body in order to get the purification of mind. Meditation is the practice of concentration [Ekagratha]. This can be done through a variety of meditation techniques. But whatever may be the method, the main purpose of meditation is to control our mind. The importance and significance of meditation has been explained earlier. Now the question is how to perform meditation? Who should perform? And the ways and means to perform meditation is very important. From children to old people, men to women everyone can practise meditation without any bar.

Regarding time and duration of practice of meditation, there is a universal tradition to perform meditation preferably in the early morning and also in the evening. But during the present busy life, most of us have little time to spare for meditation. Such being the situation one can conveniently practice meditation at the convenient interval, even at his work place. The main concept is, while performing meditation one must be free from all tensions and have control over the mind. Duration of meditation also depends upon convenience and it should preferably be between 10 to 30 minutes at a time.

The place and atmosphere selected for meditation should be, clean, calm and without any disturbance. The meditation should be performed either in Padmasana or in any other yogic posture, which is convenient to perform. From yogic science, we came to know that bodily posture helps to attain concentration for meditation. Accordingly the trunk, head and neck should be straight and erect. In Yoga Shastra the Padmasana and Siddhasana are highly recommended for meditation. The meditation is for the purpose of purification of mind and hence the place and environment should be clean and free from any disturbance.

In Dhyana yoga of **Bhagvad Gita** there are several narrations regarding direction for practice of yoga and meditation to attain the highest result. The important concepts appeared in Dhyana yoga, which is explained below.

"Let the yogin try constantly to keep the mind steady, remaining in seclusion, alone, with the mind and body controlled, free from desire, and having no possession."

The main concept of meditation is to keep the mind controlled and free from all physical and wordly interests. The place should be firm and cloth should be spread on the seat which should be convenient to practise yoga and meditation.

"Holding erect and still the body, the head, and the neck, firm, gazing on the tip of his nose, without looking around."

"Serene-minded, fearless, firm in the vow of godly life, having restrained the mind, thinking of Me, and balanced, let him sit, looking up to Me as the Supreme."

In Dhyana yoga, the perfect erection of body, gazing the nose, which helps to make the mind dwell in the self. Continued with vow of Godly life [Bramhacharya] which helps to restrain the mind from all disturbance and all deviations. The fruit of yoga as given in Dhyana yoga of **Bhagvad Gita** contains:

"Thus always keeping in the mind balanced the yogin, with the mind controlled, attain to the peace abiding in Me, which culminates in Nirvana [moksha]."

"Yoga is not possible for him who eats too much, nor for him who does not eat at all, nor for him who is addicted to too much sleep, nor for him is (ever) wakeful, O Arjuna".

"To him whose food and recreation are moderate, whose exertion in action is moderate, whose sleep and waking are moderate, to him accrues yoga which is destructive of pain."

Above verses of Dhyana yoga which refer to good eating habit, free from addictions, systematic sleeping habits, restricted food and recreation are desirable requisites for perfect yoga and meditation. Most of them start yoga and meditation with enthusiasm and after lapse of few days of practice, they discontinue the practice of meditation. This is one of the common features seen both in yoga and meditation. The practice of meditation should be regular and then only one can attain the goal. The frequent discontinuation of meditation practice will not help to control the mind perfectly. Hence it is advised, all the practitioners should perform meditation systematically and without any break. The systematic meditation helps the attainment of self. According to Sri Adishankara, the determination that "The self alone is all and nothing else exists", is the highest thought of yoga and meditation. Through such systematic practice of yoga and meditation added with dispassion, the Yogi's mind attains peace verily in the self.

Different schools explain different types of meditation. Hence the technique, procedure, and methods of practice differ from one school of thought to another. Such being the case a common or uniform system of practice cannot be prescribed. The objective of meditation is the liberation of mind from all disturbing and agitating emotions, provocations and desires. In all the meditational process, the established concept starts with meditating the favourite God with utmost concentration. Keeping an idol or a picture of any favourite deity or symbol or Srichakra will be the source of concentration.

Another important concept is focusing and concentrating on an object placed in front by closing the eyes to attain concentration of mind. This is a very commonly used method of meditation.

Another method of meditation is meditating on sound. Here chanting of mantras, epics and vedas or by hearing such Vedic mantras, one can get concentration of mind.

From various theories and interpretation we come to know that meditation helps to understand ourselves first. That is, it provides self control over mind and body. In the present disturbed environment, getting mental peace and satisfaction is very difficult. We have read in our epics and teachings of sages and saints tell us that the mind is a powerful weapon in the hands of men. That is, we can control all our physical actions through proper judgement and foresight of mind. Before whatever we want to do the immediate thoughts will first come to our mind.

It is the mind, which gives the signals for all the actions of the body. That is, the entire physical activities rely on the thoughts of the mind. Any physical ill health, pain or agony, will ultimately be sensed by the mind. Even the pleasure, happiness, sorrow and agony are all processed in the mind. So the function of mind is very important to everyone. Considering this many psychologists, scientists, sages and saints advocate that discipline of mind can be attained by meditation. Having the significance of mind control, the systematic practice of

meditation has several benefits, which are explained below.
1. Meditation helps to annihilate the mind and helps to provide liveliness to the body and mind.
2. The restlessness of mind gives scope for mental agitation, anxiety and anger. The systematic practice of meditation helps to reduce anxiety, fear and anger.
3. Controlling of mind reduces the depression of mind. We come across many young students and youths who having high ambitions in their life, get depressed when their ambitions are not materialised. In such events they will become psychologically disturbed and lose all hopes in the life. By controlling the mind through meditation, one can get rid of such depression.
4. Meditation provides systematic thinking and judging capacity and helps to develop the personality of the individual. Nowadays we have seen many industries, organisations and institutions that are providing Transcendental Meditation to its executives and managers holding key positions in the organisation. The reason is the managers and executives work under stress with responsibilities loaded on their head. The practice of meditation helps to reduce all such tensions and provides sensitivity of mind to think and judge properly in tough situations.
5. Meditation helps to provide concentration, which ultimately increases the memory power of the mind. We have seen many students who have shown dull performance in their academic persuits. In such cases, meditation provides mental effectiveness and application of intelligence.
6. From various medical studies it is found that mental stress and anxiety is the main cause of deteriorating health. Nowadays the common health problems like heart disease, high blood pressure, bronchial asthma, nervous disorders and many other diseases are aggravated by stress. Systematic practice of meditation and control of mind can reduce these problems gradually.
7. Psychological disorders which are quite common among all types of people, more particularly women [Housewives as well as working women] are entangled with several stresses and strains. Because of such stress and strain we are witnessing high rate of suicide in youths and women. This is due to lack of control over the mind. The practice of meditation helps to deter all the depression and provides self-confidence to face the tough situation.
8. We have seen an increase in number of alcoholics and drug addicts everywhere. This is mainly due to lack of control over the mind. When one who gets depressed wants to opt for instant pleasures in order to forget depression and mental tension, he starts consuming alcohol, drugs, smoking, etc. Meditation not only helps to provide control of mind but also helps to desist from such bad habits.
9. Relaxation is the main concept of meditation. The systematic and continuous practice of meditation helps to provide mental and physical peace so that one can experience utmost relaxation.

Index of Yogic Exercises/Herbal Therapy for Various Diseases

1. ACIDITY

I. Suryanamaskara: 13 times with mantras.

II. Yogasana
1. Sarvangasana (56)
2. Setubandha Sarvangasana (59)
3. Jathara Parivarthanasana (60)
4. Hanumana Valikilyasana (62)
5. Bhujangasana (70)
6. Dhanurasana (79)
7. Shirshasana (84)
8. Paschimothanasana (38)
9. Parirutha Janu Shirshasana (37)
10. Matsyendrasana (41)
11. Ardha Chakrasana (18)
12. Ardha Chandrasana (17)

III. Pranayama
1. Anuloma-Viloma
2. Chandra Bhedana
3. Ujjayi
4. Nadishodhana

IV. Herbal/Food Therapy
1. Taking watermelon in sufficient quantity reduces acidity.
2. Taking raisins/cherries regularly helps to cure acidity.
3. Taking potato, helps to reduce acidity.
4. Taking lemon juice in lukewarm water daily twice, helps to cure acidity.

2. AGEUSIA (Loss of Sense of Taste)

I. Suryanamaskara: 13 times with mantras.

II. Yogasana
1. Simhasana (29)
2. Matsyasana (30)
3. Sarvangasana (56)
4. Shirshasana (84)

III. Pranayama
1. Sitali
2. Sheethkari
3. Bhamari
4. Sadhantha
5. Ujjayi
6. Anuloma-Viloma
7. Nadishodhana

IV. Herbal/Food Therapy
1. Taking the paste of ginger added with lemon juice helps to increase the sense of taste and appetite.
2. Taking decoction of ptychotis copticum (Ajwain-omam) regularly helps to increase the appetite and sense of taste.
3. Washing the mouth with lemon juice helps to increase the sense of taste.
4. Prepare a paste with black pepper and little ginger juice. Washing the mouth with this juice helps to restore the sense of taste.

3. AMNESIA (Forgetfulness)

I. Suryanamaskara: 13 times with mantras.

II. Yogasana
1. Shirshasana (84)
2. Natarajasana (14)
3. Matsyasana (30)
4. Sarvangasana (56)
5. Karna Peedasana (97)
6. Mulabandasana (51)
7. Paschimothanasana (38)
8. Urdwa Paschimothanasana (39)
9. Sukhasana (28)
10. Veerasana (23)
11. Siddhasana (21)

12. Padmasana (20)
13. Vrikshasana (6)

III. Pranayama
1. Anuloma-Viloma
2. Ujjayi
3. Chandrabhedana
4. Suryabhedana
5. Nadishodhana

IV. Meditation

V. Herbal/Food Therapy
1. Indian pennywort [centella] is the effective remedy for forgetfulness. Taking 3 to 4 leaves of Indian pennywort early in the morning and during night will help to increase sharpness of mind and restoration of good memory.
2. Taking decoction of cumin seeds early in the morning helps to cure forgetfulness.

Note: Meditation, pranayama and yogic exercises are to be practiced regularly in order to enrich the power of mind and nervous system.

4. ANAEMIA

I. Suryanamaskara: 13 times with mantras

II. Yogasana
1. Sarvangasana (56)
2. Shirshasana (84)
3. Matsyasana (30)
4. Suptha Veerasana (24)
5. Paryankasana (25)
6. Paschimothanasana (38)
7. Matsyendrasana (41)

III. Pranayama
1. Ujjayi
2. Nadishodhana

IV. Herbal/Food Therapy
1. Taking good amount of fruits/fruit juices and dry fruits helps to cure anaemia very quickly.
2. Taking vegetables like green, leafy vegetables and other items, which are rich in iron content, helps to recover from chronic anaemia.
3. Taking unspiced brinjals helps to recover from anaemia.

5. ANOREXIA (Loss of Appetite)

I. Suryanamaskara: 13 times with mantras

II. Yogasana
1. Shirshasana (84)
2. Sarvangasana (56)
3. Matsyasana (30)
4. Paschimothanasana (38)
5. Ushtrasana (43)
6. Bhujangasana (70)
7. Simhasana (29)
8. Shalabhasana (75)
9. Dhanurasana (79)
10. Makarasana (78)

III. Pranayama
All types of Pranayama

IV. Herbal/Food Therapy
1. Taking lime juice added with ginger early in the morning cures Anorexia.
2. Taking plenty of vegetables, particularly more of cucumber, onion, and fruits helps to arrest loss of appetite.
3. Take a teaspoonful of Emblic myrobalans [Amla] with honey.

6. ARTHRITIS

I. Suryanamaskara: 6 times with mantras

II. Yogasana
1. Viparitha Karni (55)
2. Sarvangasana (56)
3. Padmasana (20)
4. Shalabhasana (75)
5. Dhanurasana (79)
6. Shirshasana (84)
7. Parshva Konasana (8)
8. Shavasana (100)

III. Pranayama
1. Anuloma-Viloma
2. Ujjayi
3. Nadishodhana

IV. Meditation

V. Herbal/Food Therapy
1. Taking decoction of Babreng seeds [Embelia ribes] regularly helps to cure arthritic pain.
2. Powder of Gigantic Swallowwort root mixed with honey is to be applied in the region of the arthritic pain.
3. Giving hot compresses on the painful joints helps to get relief from the pain.

7. APPENDICITIS

I. **Suryanamaskara:** 6 times with mantras.

II. Yogasana
1. Trikonasana (3)
2. Veerabadrasana (4)
3. Padmasana (7)
4. Ardha Padmothanasana (11)
5. Shirshasana (84)
6. Sarvangasana (56)
7. Mayurasana (33 & 34)
8. Matsyendrasana (41)
9. Veerasana (23)
10. Suptha Veerasana (24)
11. Upavishta konasana (46)
12. Hanumanasana (61)
13. Hanumana Valikilyasana (62)
14. Vibhakta Janu Shirshasana (63)

III. Pranayama
1. Anuloma-Viloma
2. Nadishodhana

IV. Herbal/Food Therapy
1. Using Eugenia Jambolana (Jamun) regularly helps to cure bleeding piles.
2. Take onion juice and mix a little honey. Taking 2-3 times a day helps to cure appendicitis.
3. Taking juice of Bengal Quince regularly helps to cure bleeding in appendicitis.
4. Decoction of Conch grass (Cynodon dactylon) helps to cure all types of piles.
5. Take a well-ripened Banana and add one teaspoonful of limejuice and honey. Taking this helps to cure appendicitis.

8. ASTHMA

I. Suryanamaskara: 13 times with mantras.

II. Yogasana
1. Viparitha Karni (55)
2. Sarvangasana (56)
3. Ushtrasana (43)
4. Suptha virasana (24)
5. Simhasana (29)
6. Bhujangasana (70)
7. Dhanurasana (79)
8. Urdwa Dhanurasana (82)
9. Tadasana (1)
10. Ardhakati Chakrasana (2)
11. Veerabhadrasana (4)
12. Shavasana (100)

III. Pranayama
1. Anuloma-Viloma
2. Ujjayi
3. Nadishodhana

IV. Herbal/Food Therapy
1. Taking juice of Grapes or Lemon gives good results in Asthma.
2. Take one teaspoonful of turmeric powder, which is to be heated and add a little honey. Taking this regularly cures bronchial asthma.
3. Take powder of piper longum (long pepper) and add a little honey. Regular use of this helps to control asthma.
4. Juice of holy basil with honey helps to cure Bronchial asthma.
5. Juice of Bengal Quince leaves with honey helps to cure asthma.

9. BALDNESS AND HAIR LOSS

I. Suryanamaskara: 13 times with mantras.

II. Yogasana
1. Shirshasana (84)
2. Matsyasana (30)
3. Sarvangasana (56)
4. Halasana (57)
5. Karna Peedasana (97)
6. Paryankasana (25)
7. Parshvothanasana (9)

8. Paschimothanasana (38)
9. Urdwa Paschimothanasana (39)
10. Ushtrasana (43)
11. Dhanurasana (79)
12. Urdwa Dhanurasana (82)
13. Makarasana (78)
14. Tittibhasana (53)
15. Tripura Harasana (15)
16. Hanumanavalikilyasana (62)
17. Rajakapothasana (72)
18. Yoganidrasana (69)
19. Purna Shalabhasana (76)
20. Laghu Vajrasana (44)

III. **Pranayama**
All types of Pranayama.

IV. **Herbal/Food therapy**
1. Take paste of opium and add a little limejuice. Apply the paste to the head and leave for 3 to 4 hours and then wash the hair. This helps to arrest hair loss.
2. Take 2 to 3 teaspoonfuls of black tea, add a little lemon juice and mix them properly and apply them on the head. After 2-3 hours of application, wash the head. This helps to cure baldness.
3. Prepare a paste from hibiscus leaves. Add a little lemon juice, mix them gently and apply over the head. Wait 2-3 hours and then wash.

10. BACKACHE

I. **Suryanamaskara:** 13 times with mantras.

II. **Yogasana**
1. All standing yogasana postures
2. Pavanamuktasana (96)
3. Matsyendrasana (41)
4. Sarvangasana (56)
5. Shirshasana (84)
6. Paschimothasana (38)
7. Janu Shirshasana (36)
8. Parirutha janushirshasana (37)
9. Ushtrasana (43)
10. Paryankasana (25)

11. Suptha Veerasana (24)
12. Chakrasana (85)
13. Bhujangasana (70)
14. Makarasana (78)
15. Dhanurasana (79 to 83)
16. Matsyasana (30)
17. Shavasana (100)

III. Pranayama
All types of Pranayama.

IV. Meditation for 10 minutes.

V. Herbal/Food Therapy
1. Application of neem oil in the region of the back and also doing massage for sometime helps to get relief from back pain.
2. Pouring cold and hot water over the back region helps to increase blood circulation and get relief from back pain.
3. Taking sufficient water, fruits and more particularly dry fruits help to tone up the body and gives relief from back pain.

Note: Performing all the standing exercises given in the book and practice of perfect standing and sitting position helps to get relief from back pain.

11. BOILS AND PUSTULES

I. Suryanamaskara

II. Yogasana
1. Shirshasana (84)
2. Sarvangasana (56)
3. Shavasana (100)

III. Herbal/Food Therapy
1. Prepare a paste from Amaranthus Spinosus (Spiny Amaranthus) leaves and add a little turmeric powder. Apply the paste over the boils.
2. Regular use of curds helps to purify the blood and in turn helps to check boils and pustules.
3. Using drumstick regularly helps to check boils. Prepare a paste from drumsticks, add a little turmeric. Mix the paste and apply over the region of boils and pustules for getting relief.
4. Take a ripe banana and make a paste by adding a few drops of lemon juice. Apply the paste on boils, this gives immediate relief.

12. COLD AND CATARRH

I. Suryanamaskara: 13 times with mantras.

II. Yogasana
1. Shirshasana (84)
2. Sarvangasana (56)
3. Yoga Nidrasana (69)
4. Paschimothanasana (38)
5. Urdwa Muka Paschimothanasana (39)
6. Upavista Konasana (46)
7. Shavasana (100)

III. Pranayama
1. Anuloma-Viloma
2. Ujjayi
3. Suryabhedana
4. Nadishodhana

IV. Meditation

V. Herbal/Food Therapy
1. Take hot water and add lemon juice. Taken twice daily gives relief from cold and catarrh.
2. Soak a few raisins (dry grapes) in water and put the same in the milk. The milk should be boiled. Take them twice daily.
3. Pineapple juice added with honey gives relief from cold.
4. Grape juice helps to act as expectorant, which helps to cure cold and cough.

13. COLIC OR GASTRALGIA

I. Suryanamaskara: 13 times with mantras.

II. Yogasana
1. Shirshasana (84)
2. Sarvangasana (56)
3. Matsyasana (30)
4. Padahastasana (7)
5. Shavasana (100)

III. Pranayama
1. Anuloma-Viloma
2. Ujjayi
3. Chandrabhedana
4. Sitali

    5. Sheethkari
    6. Bhamari
    7. Nadishodhana

IV. Herbal/Food Therapy
1. Taking juice of pomegranate daily is a good remedy for colic.
2. Add the juice of ginger to lukewarm water. Taking this juice 2 to 3 times in a day helps to cure colic.
3. Lime juice in lukewarm water taken 2-3 times in a day helps to cure colic.

14. CONSTIPATION

I. Suryanamaskara: 13 times with mantras.

II. Yogasana
1. Sarvangasana (56)
2. Shirshasana (84)
3. Paschimothanasana (38)
4. Janu Shirshasana (36)
5. Shavasana (100)

III. Pranayama
1. Anuloma-Viloma
2. Ujjayi
3. Nadishodhana

IV. Herbal/Food Therapy
1. Soak two or three figs (Ficus carica) in water for about a day. Taking the juice twice daily cures constipation.
2. The juice prepared from the leaves of Anona Squamosa (custard apple) with honey is beneficial for constipation.
3. Taking raw cucumber regularly helps to cure constipation.
4. Taking decoction of Fenugreek (trigonella foenum) regularly helps to cure constipation.

15. COUGH AND THROAT DISORDERS

I. Suryanamaskara: 13 times with mantras.

II. Yogasana
1. Simhasana (29)
2. Shirshasana (84)
3. Shalabhasana (75)
4. Dhanurasana (79)

5. Ardha Chakrasana (18)
   6. Ardha Chandrasana (17)
   7. Matsyasana (30)
   8. Paryankasana (25)
   9. Bhujangasana (70)
   10. Urdwa Dhanurasana (82)
   11. Sarvangasana (56)
   12. Shavasana (100)

III. **Pranayama**
   1. Anuloma-Viloma
   2. Ujjayi
   3. Suryabhedana
   4. Nadishodhana

IV. **Herbal/Food Therapy**
   1. Prepare a paste from piper longum (long pepper) and add a little honey. Mix the paste evenly and take 2-3 times a day, helps to cure all cough and throat disorders.
   2. Prepare a juice from holy basil (ocimum sanctum) and juice of ginger taken in equal quantity. Add a little honey and take 2-3 times a day. This helps to cure cough and throat disorders.
   3. The decoction of Liquorice roots help to cure cough and throat infections.

16. CONCENTRATION OF MIND AND ENRICHMENT OF MEMORY

I. **Suryanamaskara:** 13 times with mantras.

II. **Yogasana**
   1. Natarajasana (14)
   2. Tadasana (1)
   3. Trivikramasana (16)
   4. Trikonasana (3)
   5. Tripura Harasana (15)
   6. Vrikshasana (6)
   7. Matsyasana (30)
   8. Paryankasana (25)
   9. Sarvangasana (56)
   10. Triarngya Mukothanasana (91)
   11. Shirshasana (84)
   12. Mayurasana (33)
   13. Padmasana (20)
   14. Vrischikasana (94)

15. Paschimothanasana (38)
16. Shavasana (100)

III. Herbal/Food Therapy
Same as explained in Amnesia [Forgetfulness].

17. DIABETES

I. Suryanamaskara: 13 times with mantras

II. Yogasana
1. Shirshasana (84)
2. Sarvangasana (56)
3. Mayurasana (33)
4. Matsyendrasana (41)
5. Marichasana (40)
6. Hanumanavalikilyasana (62)
7. Bhujangasana (70)
8. Jatara Parivarthanasana (60)
9. Navasana (47)
10. Matsyasana (30)
11. Paryanakasana (25)
12. Dhanurasana (79)
13. Urdwa Dhanurasana (82)
14. Shalabhasana (78)
15. Paschimothanasana (38)

III. Pranayama
1. Anuloma-Viloma
2. Ujjayi
3. Nadishodana

IV. Herbal/Food Therapy
1. Take the juice of Emblic Myrobalans and add a little quantity of Turmeric powder and honey. Taking this for 2 to 3 times a day for about one month controls diabetes.
2. Daily taking the juice of Bengal quince (Aegle marmelos) in the early morning and at night helps to control diabetes.
3. Decoction of neem leaves helps to control diabetes.
4. Taking 8 to 10 curry leaves daily helps control diabetes.
5. The seeds of jaman (Eugenia jambolana) should be dried and powdered. Add a little turmeric powder and lime juice. Taking this 2 to 3 times daily helps to control diabetes.

18. DIARRHOEA

I. Suryanamaskara: 13 times with Mantras.

II. Yogasana
1. Shirshasana (84)
2. Sarvangasana (56)
3. Suptha Veerasana (24)
4. Shavasana (100)

III. Herbal/Food Therapy
1. Taking juice of black berry added with a little quantity of salt 2 to 3 times a day helps to check Diarrhoea.
2. Take few slices of half-ripe papaw and immerse with honey. Taking the slices early in the morning helps to check diarrhoea.
3. Taking lime juice added with little salt 2 to 3 times a day helps to cure diarrhoea. Take 6-7 cloves, immerse in a water for 6-7 hours. Taking this water helps to cure diarrhoea.

19. DIGESTIVE DISORDER

I. Suryanamaskara: 13 times with mantras.

II. Yogasana
1. All standing Yogasana Postures
2. Sarvangasana (56)
3. Shirshasana (84)
4. Matsyasana (30)
5. Mayurasana (33)
6. Paryanakasana (25)
7. Bhujangasana (70)
8. Shalabhasana (78)
9. Dhanurasana (79)
10. Ushtrasana (43)
11. Laghu Vajrasana (44)
12. Rajakapothasana (72 and 73)
13. Kurmasana (48)
14. Upavista Konasana (46)
15. Jathara Parivarthanasana (60)
16. Shavasana (100)

III. Pranayama
1. Anuloma-Viloma
2. Ujjayi
3. Nadishodana

IV. Herbal/Food Therapy
1. Juice of ginger or lemon (one teaspoonful) for 2 to 3 times a day help to cure all digestive disorders.
2. Taking lots of water helps to avoid digestive disorders.
3. Taking a decoction of caraway seeds (Ptychotis Ajowan) 2 to 3 times a day helps to cure all digestive disorders.
4. Take a few slices of papaya and add lime juice and pepper powder. Taken in little quantities 2 to 3 times a day helps to cure all the digestive problems.
5. Prepare a paste from Isabgol seeds (plantago ovata) and add a little honey. Taking this regularly will cure all digestive disorders.

20. DYSENTERY

I. Suryanamaskara: 13 times with mantras.

II. Yogasana
1. Sarvangasana (56)
2. Shirshasana (84)
3. Suptha Veerasana (24)
4. Shavasana (100)

III. Herbal/Food Therapy
1. Make a paste from a few curry leaves and add to buttermilk. Strain well and drink this 2-3 times a day. Helps to check dysentery.
2. Taking Bael fruit (unripe) daily helps to cure dysentery.
3. Take a little mango fruit and add a little curd and honey. Taking this helps to cure dysentery.
4. Taking pomegranate juice helps to reduce dysentery.

21. EAR PROBLEMS

I. Suryanamaskara: 13 times with mantras.

II. Yogasana
1. Sarvangasana (56)
2. Shirshasana (84)
3. Karna Peedasana (97)
4. Akarna Dhanurasana (83)
5. Matsyasana (30)
6. Shavasana (100)

III. Pranayama
1. Anuloma-Viloma
2. Ujjayi
3. Nadishodana

IV. **Herbal/Food Therapy**
 1. First carefully clean the ears with the good earbuds. Putting a few drops of water with vinegar to the ears 3-4 times a day clears all ear infections.
 2. Heat onion juice and allow it to cool for sometime. Put 3-4 drops of the onion juice 2-3 times in a day. Helps to control the discharge from the ears and earache.
 3. Juice of holy Basil (Tulasi) or juice of garlic can also be used as eardrops for all ear ailments.

22. ENLARGEMENT OF PROSTATE GLANDS AND SPLEEN

I. **Suryanamaskara:** 13 times with mantras.

II. **Yogasana**
 1. Sarvangasana (56)
 2. Shirshasana (84)
 3. Halasana (57)
 4. Karna Peedasana (97)
 5. Jatara Parivarthanasana (60)
 6. Uttanasana (13)
 7. Matsyendrasana (41)
 8. Kurmasana (48)
 9. Shavasana (100)

III. **Pranayama**
 1. Anuloma-Viloma
 2. Nadishodana

IV. **Herbal/Food Therapy**
 1. Taking lemon juice added with ginger regularly helps to cure enlargement of prostate glands.
 2. Make a paste from the bark of Bengal Quince. Add a few drops of honey and take the mixture 2-3 times a day.
 3. Extract the milk from unripe papaya fruit or extract milk from the papaya stem and take half a teaspoonful for 30 days. Helps to cure enlargement of prostate glands.

23. EYE DISORDERS

I. **Suryanamaskara:** 13 times with mantras.

II. **Yogasana**
 1. Shirshasana (84)
 2. Sarvangasana (56)

3. Paschimothanasana (38)
   4. Matsyasana (30)
   5. Paryankasana (25)
   6. Matsyendrasana (41)
   7. Mayurasana (33)
   8. Ushtrasana (43)
   9. Raja Kapothasana (72)
  10. Shavasana (100)

III. Pranayama
   1. Anuloma-Viloma
   2. Ujjayi
   3. Nadishodana

IV. Meditation:
Focusing the Eyes towards the tip of the nose and towards the eye brow centre for about 5 to 10 minutes.

V. Herbal/Food Therapy
   1. Washing the eyes regularly with the decoction of coriander seeds helps to increase the sharpness of the eyes. It is helpful in all the eye disorders.
   2. Juice of Emblic Myrobalan (Amla) mixed with the juice of winter cherry in equal quantity should be taken internally 2 times daily. Helps to increase the sharpness of eyes.
   3. Taking decoction of Triphala internally as well as washing the eyes with Triphala decoction helps to cure all the eye problems.
   4. Taking daily the juice of raw onion mixed with honey have many advantages for eye disorders.

Note: Avoid exposure of eyes to dust, smoke or very bright light. Reading in inadequate light, smoking, drinking, unlimited sex will cause eye disorders. Washing the eyes daily with clean water, taking healthy diet of milk, fruits and vegetables are recommended. Raw carrots, almonds are quite helpful in eye disorders.

24. EPILEPSY

I. Suryanamaskara: 13 times with mantras.

II. Yogasana
   1. Sarvangasana (56)
   2. Shirshasana (84)
   3. Halasana (57)
   4. Paschimothanasana (38)
   5. Matsyasana (30)

      6. Paryankasana (25)
      7. Suptha Veerasana (24)
      8. Shavasana (100)

III. Pranayama
1. Anuloma-Viloma
2. Ujjayi
3. Nadishodhana

IV. Herbal/Food Therapy
1. Extract juice from the leaves of Indian pennywort (Centella) and add a little honey. Take the juice internally twice daily. It is an effective remedy for epilepsy.
2. Paste of Emblic Myrobalans mixed with curds and then heated for some minutes, should be massaged over the foerhead as well as the crown of the head. Helps to cure epilepsy.
3. The juice of white onion used as nose drops helps to cure epilepsy.
4. Giving grape juice thrice a day helps to avoid epilepsy.

Precaution: When epilepsy attacks the precaution is to pour cold water on the face and place any iron metal, which should touch the body.

25. EXHAUSTION AND FATIGUE

I. Suryanamaskara: 5 to 6 times with mantras.

II. Yogasana
1. Sarvangasana (56)
2. Shirshasana (84)
3. Uttanasana (13)
4. Tadasana (1)
5. Shavasana (100)

III. Pranayama
1. Anuloma-Viloma
2. Nadishodhana

IV. Herbal/Food Therapy
1. Take lemon juice and add sugar and salt. Taking this 2 to 3 times daily provides energy and strength.
2. Consuming orange juice 3 to 4 times a day helps to reduce fatigue.
3. Taking plenty of water as well as fruit juices helps to reduce exhaustion and fatigue.
4. Juice of black berry taken 2 to 3 times a day helps to reduce exhausticn and fatigue.

26. GOUT

I. Suryanamaskara: 13 times with mantras.

II. Yogasana
1. All standing yogasana Postures
2. Shirshasana (84)
3. Sarvangasana (56)
4. Gomukhasana (42)
5. Matsyendrasana (41)
6. Matsyasana (30)
7. Paryankasana (25)
8. Yoganidrasana (69)
9. Dhanurasana (79)
10. Paschimothanasana (38)
11. Shavasana (100)

III. Pranayama
1. Anuloma-Viloma
2. Nadishodhana

IV. Herbal/Food Therapy
1. Mixture of lime juice and coconut oil should be applied on the swollen joints. Gives immediate relief.
2. Grind ginger and make a paste. Add a little drops of castor oil and Camphor and apply it to the affected joints.
3. Extract Garlic oil from garlic and apply the same to the affected joints. Gives instant relief.

27. HALITOSIS (Bad Breath)

I. Suryanamaskara: 13 times with mantras.

II. Yogasana
1. Shirshasana (84)
2. Sarvangasana (56)
3. Simhasana (29)
4. Matsyendrasana (41)
5. Matsyasana (30)
6. Paryankasana (25)
7. Jataraparivartanasana (60)
8. Paschimothanasana (38)
9. Shavasana (100)

III. Pranayama
1. Anuloma Viloma
2. Nadishodhana
3. Ujjayi
4. Sitali
5. Bhamari

IV. Herbal/Food Therapy
1. Chewing cloves or ginger helps to get rid of halitosis (bad breath)
2. Chewing fennel seeds or leaves of holy basil or cardamom helps to cure bad breath.

28. HEADACHE

I. Suryanamaskara: 13 times with mantras

II. Yogasana
1. Shirshasana (84)
2. Sarvangasana (56)
3. Halasana (57)
4. Matsyendrasana (41)
5. Matsyasana (30)
6. Paryankasana (25)
7. Uttanasana (13)
8. Dhanurasana (79)
9. Paschimothanasana (38)
10. Kurmasana (45)
11. Shavasana (100)

III. Pranayama
1. Anuloma-Viloma
2. Nadishodhana
3. Ujjayi

IV. Herbal/Food Therapy
1. Application of paste prepared from the leaves of the cashew nut on forehead.
2. Taking well ripened apple added with a little salt early in the morning on empty stomach.
3. Place the hot water pad on the back of the neck and then massage the neck and shoulder. Gives instant relief.
4. Juice of ginger added with equal quantity of lemon juice. Massage the solution on the forehead.

Note: Headache may be caused due to indigestion, constipation, nervous weakness, eyestrain, mental tension, blood pressure etc. The reason for headache has to be identified first before taking any treatment. Taking meals hurriedly, sleeplessness, over sex, too much talking, visual strains are the reasons for headache and these should be avoided.

29. HEAT EXHAUSTION AND HEAT STROKE

I. Suryanamaskara: 13 times with mantras.

II. Yogasana
1. All standing Yogasana Postures
2. Shirshasana (84)
3. Sarvangasana (56)
4. Gomukhasana (42)
5. Matsyendrasana (41)
6. Matsyasana (30)
7. Paryankasana (25)
8. Yoganidrasana (69)
9. Dhanurasana (79)
10. Paschimothanasana (38)
11. Shavasana (100)

III. Pranayama
1. Anuloma-Viloma
2. Nadishodhana
3. Ujjayi
4. Sitali
5. Sheetkari
6. Bhamari

IV. Meditation

V. Herbal/Food Therapy
1. Taking the juice of sweet orange thrice a day.
2. Taking juice of lemon added with black pepper twice a day.
3. Taking one full cup of curd added with Asafoetida twice daily.
4. Juice extracted from coriander leaves twice daily.
5. Putting cold bandage/cold compresses on forehead and wrapping the cold cloth on the entire body helps to avoid all the problems arising due to heat stroke.
6. Taking sugarcane juice reduces exhaustion due to heat.

30. HEART DISEASES

   I. **Suryanamaskara:** 1 to 2 times with mantras.

  II. **Yogasana**
    1. Uttanasana (13)
    2. Veerasana (23)
    3. Suptha Veerasana (24)
    4. Bhujangasana (70)
    5. Paschimothanasana (38)
    6. Janu Shirshasana (36)
    7. Padmasana (20)
    8. Vajrasana (22)
    9. Gomukhasana (42)
   10. Shavasana (100)

 III. **Pranayama**
    1. Anuloma-Viloma without retention (kumbaka)
    2. Ujjayi without retention (kumbaka)
    3. Nadishodana without retention (kumbaka)

 IV. **Meditation**
   For about 10 to 15 minutes

  V. **Herbal/Food Therapy**
    1. Taking honey daily in lukewarm water prevents heart diseases.
    2. Decoction of winter cherry (withania somnifera) with a few drops of lemon juice. Take the juice twice daily.
    3. Take equal amount of juice extracted from conch grass and Arjuna Myrobalan and add honey to the mixture. Take the juice twice daily.
    4. Juice extracted from Indian Pennywort (Centella) taken twice daily.

Note: Avoid drinking, smoking, and excessive sex. Reduce weight and maintain good food habits. Take enough quantity of fresh and dry fruits which have the quality to strengthen the heart.

31. HYPERTENSION (High Blood Pressure)

   I. **Suryanamaskara:** 3 to 4 times with mantras.

  II. **Yogasana**
    1. Tadasana (1)
    2. Natarajasana (14)
    3. Uttanasana (13)
    4. Halasana (57)
    5. Paschimothanasana (38)
    6. Shavasana (100)

III. Herbal/Food Therapy
1. Take a teaspoonful of Sarpagandha powder (Rauwolfia serpantina) along with honey 3 times a day.
2. Take two teaspoonfuls of raw onion juice added with honey twice, daily.
3. Chewing about 5g of fennel seeds (foeniculation capillaecum) daily in the night reduces high blood pressure.
4. One teaspoonful of amla powder (Phyllanthus Emelica) added with honey, taken daily cures high blood pressure.

Note: Emotions, mental worries are likely to increase Hypertension. Keep the mind calm and cool. Reduce weight and stop taking fatty foods, salt and saturated foods. Smoking and drinking must be stopped.

32. HERNIA

I. Suryanamaskara: 13 times with mantras

II. Yogasana
1. Sarvangasana (56)
2. Shirshasana (84)
3. Baddha Konasana (26)
4. Pada Hasthasana (7)
5. Navasana (47)
6. Dhanurasana (79)
7. Paschimothanasana (38)
8. Shavasana (100)

III. Herbal/Food Therapy
1. Prepare starch from rice and keep it for about a day. When the starch is fermented, prepare a paste from the root/stem of gigantic swallowwort (calotrapis Gigenta) and then mix with the starch. Taking this mixture helps to cure hernia.
2. Take Cumin seed and Fennel seed in equal quantity and powder the mixture. Add castor oil and apply the same on the hernia affected region.

33. HUNCH BACK

I. Suryanamaskara: 13 times with mantras.

II. Yogasana
1. All standing yogasana postures
2. Bhujangasana (57)

3. Ushtrasana (43)
   4. Baddha Konasana (26)
   5. Paschimothanasana (38)
   6. Setubanda Sarvangasana (59)
   7. Matsyasana (30)
   8. Sarvangasana (56)
   9. Hanumanasana (61)
   10. Hanumana valikilyasana (62)
   11. Dhanurasana (79)
   12. Yoga Nidrasana (69)
   13. Pincha Mayurasana (92)
   14. Vrischikasana (94)
   15. Gomukhasana (42)
   16. Makarasana (78)
   17. Paryankasana (25)
   18. Shavasana (100)

Note: Perfect walking style, firmness while standing and sitting position and exercise which involves extensive stretch on the back will help to get rid of hunch back. Here the more important point is that one should remember that the hunchback is not a disease but it is a wrong practice adopted by an individual. To get rid of the wrong practice one should make a determination.

34. HYSTERIA

I. Suryanamaskara: 13 times with mantras.

II. Yogasana
   1. Sarvangasana (56)
   2. Shirshasana (36)
   3. Matsyasana (30)
   4. Matsyendrasana (41)
   5. Halasana
   6. Shavasana

III. Pranayama
   1. Anuloma-Viloma
   2. Ujjayi
   3. Nadishodana

IV. Meditation

V. Herbal/Food Therapy
1. Powder of Emblic Myrobalans mixed with curds should be massaged over the forehead and also be taken internally twice daily.

2. Prepare a paste from Indian Pennywort and add honey. Take the mixture twice daily.

Note: Meditation will help to reduce the disease considerably.

35. HYPOTENSION (Low Blood Pressure)

I. Suryanamaskara: 13 times with mantras.

II. Yogasana
1. Tadasana (1)
2. Natarajasana (14)
3. Uttanasana (13)
4. Halasana (57)
5. Paschimothanasana (38)
6. Shavasana (100)

III. Herbal/Food Therapy
1. Taking nutritious foods, which contain carbohydrates and proteins like dry fruits, banana, apple, grapes, etc. help to provide strength to the body.
2. Daily taking little quantity of conch grass [Cynodon Dactylon] helps to cure hypotension.

Note: Avoid vigorous exercise, excessive sex, taking alcohol, tobacco and smoking must be avoided.

36. IMPOTENCY

I. Suryanamaskara: 13 times with mantras.

II. Yogasana
1. Viparitha Karni (55)
2. Halasana (57)
3. Baddha Konasana (26)
4. Paschimothanasana (38)
5. Setubanda Sarvangasana (59)
6. Matsyasana (30)
7. Sarvangasana (56)
8. Hanumanasana (56)
9. Dhanurasana (79)
10. Yoganidrasana (69)
11. Shavasana (100)

III. Pranayama
1. Anuloma-Viloma

    2. Ujjayi
    3. Nadishodhana
  IV. **Meditation**
   For about 10 minutes.
  V. **Herbal/Food Therapy**
    1. Decoction of Emblic Myrobalans (Amla) taken internally daily twice is very effective in impotency.
    2. Taking powder of holy basil seed with honey 3 times daily reduces impotency.
    3. The milk extracted from the stem of banyan tree added with honey taken 3-4 times daily have a definite cure for impotency.

Note : Smoking, alcoholism, indulging in unnatural sex and psychological emotions are the prime causes for inpotency. The perfect and regular practice of yogic exercise, meditation and pranayama helps to cure impotency.

37. INDIGESTION (Dyspepsia)

  I. **Suryanamaskara:** 13 times with mantras.
  II. **Yogasana**
    1. Shirshasana (84)
    2. Sarvangasana (56)
    3. Jatari Parivarthanasana (60)
    4. All standing Yogasana Postures
    5. Matsyendrasana (41)
    6. Navasana (47)
    7. Yoga Nidhrasana (69)
    8. Bhujangasana (70)
    9. Shalabhasana (78)
    10. Dhanurasana (79)
    11. Shavasana (100)
  III. **Pranayama**
    1. Anuloma-Viloma
    2. Ujjayi
    3. Nadishodana

Note: Consumption of enough water and avoiding hard foods, oily foods, chillies, and salt, helps in speedy recovery.

  IV. **Herbal/Food Therapy**
    1. Boil water with lemon juice and take the juice 4-5 times.
    2. Taking well ripened banana along with a pinch of cardamon powder while sleeping helps to cure indigestion.

3. Taking the paste of ginger added with honey for 2-3 times.
4. Decoction of ajawain (Bishop seed-ptychotis copticum) administered 3-4 times daily gets good relief.
5. Paste of Bengal quince (Aegle marmelos) added with honey should be taken 2 times a day for about a week.

38. INFLUENZA

I. Suryanamaskara: 13 times with mantras.

II. Yogasana
1. All standing postures
2. Sarvangasana (56)
3. Shirshasana (84)
4. Matsyasana (30)
5. Paryankasana (25)
6. Shavasana (100)

III. Pranayama
1. Anuloma-Viloma
2. Ujjayi
3. Nadishodhana

IV. Meditation

V. Herbal/Food Therapy
1. Juice of ginger and holy basil mixed with honey is to be taken twice daily, helps to cure influenza.
2. Take well-ripened banana and cut into slices, add pepper powder and honey. Take this early in the morning for 15 days.
3. Juice of ginger added with honey taken twice daily helps to cure influenza.

39. INSOMNIA (Sleeplessness)

I. Suryanamaskara

II. Yogasana
1. Shirshasana (84)
2. Sarvangasana (58)
3. Paschimothanasana (58)
4. Uttanasana (13)
5. Shavasana (100)

III. **Pranayama**
 1. Anuloma-Viloma
 2. Ujjayi
 3. Nadishodhana

IV. **Meditation**

V. **Herbal/Food Therapy**
 1. Powders of Indian Pennywort (Centella), Emblic Myrobalans (Phyllanthus Emelica) and Bengal Quince (Aegle Marmelos) mixed in equal quantity and taken in doses of 1 teaspoonful 3 times daily with honey.
 2. Taking paste of Emblic Myrobalans (Amla) regularly while going to bed helps to cure sleeplessness.
 3. Take hot water in a vessel and place both the feet in it. Place the wet towel (immersed in cold water) on the forehead, and stay for 10-15 minutes before going to bed. This not only cures sleeplessness but is also effective for mental, eyes and heart problems.

Note: For sleeplessness do not take pills or medicines. Avoid coffee, tea, smoking, drinking or other intoxications. Consumption of enough water and fruits is more helpful in this problem. Massaging, oil bathing, listening to music while going to bed is helpful. Meditation is very useful in sleeplessness.

40. INTESTINAL PARASITES/PROBLEMS

I. **Suryanamaskara:** 13 times with mantras.

II. **Yogasana**
 1. Shirshasana (84)
 2. Sarvangasana (56)
 3. Halasana (57)
 4. Karna Peedasana (97)
 5. Matsyasana (30)
 6. Paryankasana (25)
 7. Paschimothanasana (38)
 8. Matsyendrasana (41)
 9. Shavasana (100)

III. **Pranayama**
 1. Anuloma-Viloma
 2. Ujjayi
 3. Nadishodhana

IV. **Herbal/Food Therapy**
 1. Juice of Indian wild pepper mixed with curds taken in the early morning clears the intestinal worms.

2. Juice extracted from the root of pomegranate is very effective treatment for intestinal parasites.
3. Juice of pumpkin taken twice daily for one week clears all the intestinal worms.

41. JAUNDICE

I. Suryanamaskara: 13 times with mantras.

II. Yogasana
1. Sarvangasana (56)
2. Shirshasana (84)
3. Matsyasana (36)
4. Dhanurasana (79)
5. Shavasana (100)

III. Pranayama
1. Anuloma-Viloma
2. Ujjayi
3. Nadishodhana
4. Shitali
5. Sheethkari
6. Bhamari

IV. Herbal/Food Therapy
1. One teaspoonful of turmeric mixed with pure curds and kept for a day. Taking this mixture daily early in the morning cures jaundice.
2. Taking juice of sugarcane daily is highly beneficial.
3. Paste of emblic myrobalans added with lemon juice. Take the mixture twice daily.
4. Soak few leaves of Henna in water overnight. Drinking the decoction of Henna water early in the morning cures jaundice.

42. KIDNEY PROBLEMS

I. Suryanamaskara: 13 times with mantras.

II. Yogasana
1. Shirshasana (84)
2. Sarvangasana (56)
3. Hanumana Valikilyasana (62)
4. Natarajasana (14)
5. Tripura Harasana (15)
6. Shalabhasana (74)

7. Viparitha Shalabhasana (77)
   8. Purna Dhanurasana (81)
   9. Ganda Berundasana (90)
   10. Triangya Mukothanasana (91)
   11. Yoga Nidhrasana (69)
   12. Omkarasana (66)
   13. Matsyendrasana (41)
   14. Parirutha Janu Shirshasana (37)
   15. Vrischikasana (94 & 95)
   16. Shavasana (100)

III. Pranayama
   1. Anuloma-Viloma
   2. Ujjayi
   3. Nadishodana

IV. Herbal/Food Therapy
   1. Taking enough quantity of water/tender coconut helps to cure various kidney problems.
   2. Mango and pineapple juice is very helpful in curing weakness of kidneys.
   3. For urination by drops, the juice of raisins is helpful.
   4. The juice extracted from pumpkin helps to cure pains during urination.
   5. Immerse 2-3 figs in water for 8-10 hours. Take the juice daily. Helps to cure kidney stones.
   6. Take the paste of Emblic Myrobalans and a little honey. Taking this for 2-3 times a day helps to cure passing of blood in urine.
   7. Taking honey regularly helps to cure excess urination.

43. LEG PAIN

I. Suryanamaskara: 13 times with mantras.

II. Yogasana
   1. All standing Yogasana Postures
   2. Hanumanasana (61)
   3. Hanumana Valikilyasana (62)
   4. Padmasana (20)
   5. Vajrasana (22)
   6. Veerasana (23)
   7. Supthaveerasana (24)
   8. Samakonasana (52)
   9. Baddha konasana (26)

10. Mulabandasana (51)
   11. Kurmasana (45)
   12. Upavista Konasana (46)
   13. Ekapada Shaynadanda Ekahasta Mayurasana (35)
   14. Shavasana (100)

III. Herbal/Food Therapy
   1. Heat coconut oil mixed with garlic for some time and allow to cool. Rub it mildly over the leg.
   2. Immerse the legs in hot and cold water alternatively. Helps reduce leg pain.
   3. Add a little vinegar and salt to the water. Wash the legs with this water. Helps to reduce leg pain considerably.

44. LIVER PROBLEMS

I. Suryanamaskara: 13 times with mantras.

II. Yogasana
   1. Shirshasana (84)
   2. Sarvangasana (56)
   3. Hanumana Valikilyasana (62)
   4. Natarajasana (14)
   5. Tripura Harasana (15)
   6. Shalabhasana (78)
   7. Viparitha Shalabhasana (78)
   8. Purna Dhanurasana (81)
   9. Gandabherundasana (90)
   10. Triangya Mukothanasana (91)
   11. Yoga Nidhrasana (69)
   12. Omkarasana (66)
   13. Matsyendrasana (41)
   14. Parirutha Janu Shirshasana (37)
   15. Vrischikasana (94 & 95)
   16. Shavasana (100)

III. Pranayama
   1. Anuloma-Viloma
   2. Ujjayi
   3. Nadishodana

IV. Herbal/Food Therapy
   1. Juice of lemon mixed with hot water taken 2-3 times daily effectively cures liver problems.

2. Take few slices of pineapple, which are to be immersed in honey for 3-4 days. Taking the slices of the pineapple 4 times a day cures all the liver complaints.
3. Taking juice of fig is good for liver complaints.
4. Taking sugarcane juice frequently helps to cure liver problems.
5. Prepare a paste from Emblic Myrobalans and take it 3-4 times a day. Helps to cure all the liver problems.

45. MIGRAINE
   I. **Suryanamaskara:** 13 times with mantras.
   II. **Yogasana**
      1. Shirshasana (84)
      2. Sarvangasana (56)
      3. Uttanasana (13)
      4. Paschimothanasana (38)
      5. Padmasana (20)
      6. Shavasana (100)
   III. **Herbal/Food Therapy**
      1. Taking juice of grapes daily is effective for migraine.
      2. Using good quantity of Bengal gram (cicer aricentinum) regularly gives relief from migraine headache.
      3. Applying the paste of cloves on forehead and around the nose helps to cure migraine.
      4. Prepare a paste from neem leaves. Add a little castor oil. Heat mildly and apply on forehead. Gives instant relief from migraine headache.

46. MUSCULAR AND BODY PAIN
   I. **Suryanamaskara:** 13 times with mantras.
   II. **Yogasana**
      1. Sarvangasana (56)
      2. Shirshasana (84)
      3. Halasana (57)
      4. Samakonasana (52)
      5. Kurmasana (45)
      6. Bhujangasana (70)
      7. Shavasana (100)
   III. **Herbal/Food Therapy**
      1. Extract oil from lemon grass (Citrus Auratifolia) and apply to the affected area. This gives immediate relief.

2. Prepare paste from tamarind fruit and add a little turmeric to the paste. Apply the paste on the affected area, I gives good relief.
3. The neem oil extracted from neem leaves is to be applied over the affected parts for immediate relief.
4. Extract juice from garlic and add a little turmeric powder. Apply the juice over the affected parts for immediate relief.
5. Taking the juice of Tinospora Cordifolia regularly helps to get relief from body and muscular pain.

47. NERVOUS PROBLEMS

I. **Suryanamaskara:** 13 times with mantras.

II. **Yogasana**
1. Shirshasana (84)
2. Halasana (57)
3. Badda Konasana (26)
4. Samakonasana (52)
5. Kurmasana (48)
6. Matsyendrasana (41)
7. Paryankasana (25)
8. Paschimothanasana (38)
9. Hanumanasana (61)
10. Mulabandasana (51)
11. Sarvangasana (56)
12. Bhujangasana (70)
13. Dhanurasana (79)
14. Shavasana (100)

III. **Pranayama**
1. Anuloma-Viloma
2. Ujjayi
3. Nadishodana

IV. **Herbal/Food Therapy**
1. Take a few raisins and soak them in water. In the morning take that juice mixed with a little honey. Taking this regularly cures all the nervous problems.
2. Grape as well as fig juice helps to tone up the nervous system of the body.
3. A decoction prepared from Tinospora Cordifolia and decoction of Abrus precatorius (country liquorice) mixed in equal quantity taken regularly helps to cure all the nervous disorders.
4. Dry fruits like dates, almonds etc. also help to cure nervous problems.

48. PARALYSIS

I. Suryanamaskara: 13 times with mantras.

II. Yogasana
1. Shirshasana (84)
2. Halasana (57)
3. Suptha Veerasana (24)
4. Paschimothanasana (38)
5. Sarvangasana (56)
6. Bhujangasana (70)
7. Dhanurasana (79)
8. Shavasana (100)

III. Pranayama
1. Anuloma-Viloma
2. Ujjayi
3. Nadishodana

IV. Herbal/Food Therapy
1. Taking decoction of Heart leaves (tinospora cordifolia) regularly helps to cure paralysis.
2. Prepare a paste from Acorus calamas (Sweet Flag) stem, add a little honey. Taking this help to cure paralysis.
3. Daily consuming Indian pennywort (centella) helps to tone up the nervous system and also promotes fast recovery from paralysis.

49. OBESITY

I. Suryanamaskara: 13 times with mantras.

II. Yogasana
1. Shirshasana (84)
2. Halasana (57)
3. Baddha Konasana (26)
4. Samakonasana (52)
5. Kurmasana (48)
6. Matsyendrasana (41)
7. Paryankasana (25)
8. Paschimothanasana (38)
9. Hanumanasana (61)
10. Mulabandasana (51)
11. Sarvangasana (56)
12. Bhujangasana (70)
13. Dhanurasana (79)

    14. Mayurasana (33)
    15. Pincha Mayurasana (92)
    16. Chakrasana (85)
    17. Shavasana (100)

III. Pranayama
    1. Anuloma-Viloma
    2. Ujjayi
    3. Nadishodana

IV. Herbal/Food Therapy
    1. Taking lemon juice with honey in the morning and at night regularly helps to arrest obesity.
    2. Taking the powder of Amla (Emblic myrobalans) with honey helps to reduce the body weight.
    3. Taking raw onion regularly helps to reduce cholesterol in the body and also helps to reduce the fatness of the body.
    4. Taking regularly the paste of conch grass (cynodon dactylon) with honey helps to reduce the body weight.

50. RHEUMATIC FEVER

I. Suryanamaskara: 13 times with mantras.

II. Yogasana
    1. Shirshasana (84)
    2. Halasana (57)
    3. Suptha Veerasana (24)
    4. Paschimothanasana (38)
    5. Sarvangasana (56)
    6. Bhujangasana (70)
    7. Dhanurasana (79)
    8. Shavasana (100)

III. Pranayama
    1. Anuloma-Viloma
    2. Ujjayi
    3. Nadishodana

IV. Herbal/Food Therapy
    1. Taking lemon juice twice a day helps to get relief from sickness of rheumatic fever.
    2. Powder of fenugreek and conch grass (cynodon Dactylon) mixed with honey taken twice daily helps to cure Rheumatic pain.
    3. Taking fruits like grapes, apples, mangoes, oranges, helps to get relief from pains due to rheumatic fever.

51. TOOTHACHE

I. Suryanamaskara: 13 times with mantras.

II. Yogasana
1. Simhasana (29)
2. Sarvangasana (56)
3. Matsyasana (30)
4. Paryankasana (25)
5. Shirshasana (84)
6. Paschimothanasana (38)
7. Shavasana (100)

III. Pranayama
1. Anuloma-Viloma
2. Ujjayi
3. Nadishodana
4. Shitali
5. Sadhantha
6. Bhamari

IV. Herbal/Food Therapy
1. Juice of holy basil (ocimum sanctum) applied to the aching tooth gives immediate relief.
2. Prepare a paste from Emblic myrobalans (Amla) and gargle daily twice or thrice with that paste.
3. Take a little lime juice and add a little quantity of pure lime and jaggery. Mix them in order to make a paste. Apply the paste to the gums and tooth.
4. Gargling the decoction of guava leaves twice or thrice daily.
5. Application of clove oil on gums and teeth gives immediate relief.
6. Chew one or two cashew leaves.

52. TONSILLITIS

I. Suryanamaskara: 1-3 times with mantras.

II. Yogasana
1. Shirshasana (84)
2. Yoganidrasana (69)
3. Matsyasana (30)
4. Kurmasana (48)
5. Ardha Matsyendrasana (41)
6. Paryankasana (25)

  7. Paschimothanasana (38)
  8. Marichasana (40)
  9. Sarvangasana (56)
  10. Bhujangasana (70)
  11. Dhanurasana (79)
  12. Shavasana (100)

III. Pranayama
  1. Anuloma-Viloma
  2. Ujjayi
  3. Nadishodana

IV. Herbal/Food Therapy
  1. Gargle warm salt water daily 3 or 4 times.
  2. Take the juice of black berry (eugenia jambolana) and add a little honey. Take the juice twice daily.

Note: Avoid hot, spicy food, chillies, food articles kept in the refrigerator, sour items and fried food.

53. STERILITY

I. Suryanamaskara: 1-3 times with mantras.

II. Yogasana
  1. Shirshasana (84)
  2. Halasana (57)
  3. Baddha Konasana (26)
  4. Kurmasana (48)
  5. Ardha Matsyendrasana (41)
  6. Paryankasana (25)
  7. Paschimothanasana (38)
  8. Mulabandasana (51)
  9. Sarvangasana (56)
  10. Bhujangasana (70)
  11. Dhanurasana (79)
  12. Upavista Konasana (46)
  13. Kandasana (49)
  14. Shavasana (100)

III. Pranayama
  1. Anuloma-Viloma
  2. Ujjayi
  3. Nadishodhana

IV. Herbal/Food Therapy
1. Four teaspoonfuls of onion juice, one teaspoonful of honey and half teaspoonful of ghee mixed together. This mixture is to taken daily in the morning before taking food.
2. Powder of Emblic Myrobalans (Amla) added with honey to be taken one teaspoonful daily.

Note: Smoking, drinking and excessive sex must be avoided.

54. SEXUAL VIGOUR

I. Suryanamaskara: 13 times with mantras.

II. Yogasana
1. Sarvangasana (56)
2. Bhujangasana (70)
3. Shalabhasana (75)
4. Paschimothanasana (38)
5. Shirshasana (84)
6. Dhanurasana (79)
7. Shavasana (100)

III. Pranayama
1. Anuloma-Viloma
2. Ujjayi
3. Nadishodana

IV. Meditation

V. Herbal/Food Therapy
1. Paste of linseed leaves mixed with curds taken daily helps to increase sexual vigour and increase of semen.
2. The decoction of peepul leaves helps to increase sexual vigour.
3. Taking black gram (phaseolus roxburghii) regularly helps to increase sexual vigour.
4. Taking fruits like mangoes, dates, banana, grapes etc. helps to maintain the sexual vigour.

55. TUBERCULOSIS

Suryanamaskara, Pranayama and Meditation help to ease the physical and mental discomfort that arises due to tuberculosis. Added to this, performing simple yogic exercise without getting physically strained helps in speedy recovery from tuberculosis.

I. Herbal/Food Therapy
1. Juice of malabar nut (Adhatoda vasaka) added with honey taken 3-4 times daily helps to cure early stage of TB.
2. Taking papaya fruit added with honey for 2-3 months.
3. Paste of garlic added with honey taken internally helps cure TB.
4. Powder of bengal quince and winter cherry taken in equal quantity added with honey, helps to check the progress of TB.
5. Guavas and Colocynth (Indrayan) fruits are very helpful in curing TB.

Note: Taking early precaution is very essential. Keeping clean surroundings, good environment should be maintained. Good healthy diet, plenty of pulses, fruits and milk helps in speedy recovery from TB.

56. TUMOURS OR SORES IN UTERUS/STOMACH

I. Suryanamaskara: 13 times with mantras.

II. Yogasana
1. Sarvangasana (56)
2. Shirshasana (84)
3. Matsyasana (30)
4. Paryankasana (25)
5. Paschimothanasana (38)
6. Shavasana (100)

III. Pranayama
1. Anuloma-Viloma
2. Ujjayi
3. Nadishodana
4. Bhamari

IV. Herbal/Food Therapy
1. Boil water with neem leaves. Allow to cool and wash the vaginal organs with neem water.
2. Taking the powder of Emblic Myrobalans (Amla) with honey regularly will be highly beneficial.
3. Washing the vaginal organs with the decoction prepared from the leaves of Ashoka tree (Saraca India).

9

Yogic Exercises for Special Persons

1. YOGIC EXERCISES FOR MUSICIANS AND ARTISTS

    I. **Suryanamaskara:** 13 times with mantras.

   II. **Yogasana**
      1. Sarvangasana (56)
      2. Shirshasana (84)
      3. Simhasana (29)
      4. Angustasana (48)
      5. Matsyasana (30)
      6. Paryankasana (25)
      7. Vajrasana (22)
      8. Suptha Veerasana (24)
      9. Mayurasana (33 & 34)
     10. Setubanda Sarvangasana (59)
     11. Vrischikasana (94 & 95)
     12. Hanumanasana (61)
     13. Mulabandasana (51)
     14. Makarasana (78)
     15. Shalabhasana (74)
     16. Shavasana (100)

  III. **Pranayama**
      1. Anuloma-Viloma
      2. Ujjayi
      3. Nadishodana

  IV. **Meditation**

2. YOGIC EXERCISES FOR FARMERS

I. Suryanamaskara: 5 to 6 times with mantras.

II. Yogasana
1. Shirshasana (84)
2. Sarvangasana (56)
3. Matsyasana (30)
4. Padmasana (20)
5. Vajrasana (22)
6. Suptha Veerasana (24)
7. Shavasana (100)

III. Pranayama
1. Anulcma-Viloma
2. Ujjayi
3. Nadishodhana

IV. Meditation

3. YOGIC EXERCISES FOR PREGNANT WOMEN

I. Yogasana
1. Badda Konasana (26)
2. Padmasana (20)
3. Tadasana (1)
4. Ardhakati Chakrasana (2)
5. Vajrasana (22)
6. Suptha Veerasana (24)
7. Shavasana (100)

II. Pranayama
1. Anuloma-Viloma
2. Ujjayi
3. Nadishodana

III. Meditation

4. YOGIC EXERCISES FOR AGED PEOPLE

I. Suryanamaskara: 3 to 4 times with mantras.

II. Yogasana
1. Tadasana (1)
2. Trikonasana (3)

3. Ardhakati Chakrasana (2)
4. Uttanasana (13)
5. Simhasana (29)
6. Padmasana (20)
7. Suptha Veerasana (24)
8. Bhujangasana (70)
9. Shalabhasana (74)
10. Dhanurasana (79)
11. Urdwa Dhanurasana (81)
12. Sarvangasana (56)
13. Shirshasana (84)
14. Shavasana (100)

III. Pranayama
1. Anuloma-Viloma
2. Ujjayi
3. Nadishodana

IV. Meditation

5. YOGIC EXERCISES FOR ARTISTS AND CRAFTSMEN

I. Suryanamaskara: 13 times with mantras.

II. Yogasana
1. Mayurasana (33)
2. Paryankasana (25)
3. Angustasana (48)
4. Sarvangasana (56)
5. Shirshasana (84)
6. Mulabandasana (51)
7. Vajrasana (22)
8. Padmasana (20)
9. Pincha Mayurasana (92)
10. Shavasana (100)

III. Pranayama
1. Anuloma-Viloma
2. Ujjayi
3. Nadishodana

IV. Meditation

6. YOGIC EXERCISES FOR STUDENTS

I. Suryanamaskara: 13 times with mantras.

II. Yogasana
1. All standing Yogasana Postures
2. Sarvangasana (56)
3. Shirshasana (84)
4. Matsyasana (30)
5. Paryankasana (25)
6. Ushtrasana (43)
7. Lagu Vajrasana (44)
8. Raja Kapothasana (72)
9. Hanumanasana (61)
10. Sama Konasana (52)
11. Urdwa Dhanurasana (82)
12. Dhanurasana (79)
13. Bhujangasana (70)
14. Mayurasana (33)
15. Halasana (57)
16. Karma Peedasana (97)
17. Kurmasana (48)
18. Upavista Konasana (46)
19. Mulabandasana (51)
20. Shavasana (100)

III. Pranayama
1. Anuloma-Viloma
2. Ujjayi
3. Nadishodana

IV. Meditation

7. YOGIC EXERCISES FOR EXECUTIVES AND WORKING PROFESSIONALS

I. Suryanamaskara: 5 to 6 times with mantras.

II. Yogasana
1. Tadasana (1)
2. Trikonasana (3)
3. Ardhakati Chakrasana (2)
4. Uttanasana (13)
5. Padmasana (20)
6. Matsyasana (30)

    7. Sarvangasana (56)
    8. Vajrasana (22)
    9. Shirshasana (84)
    10. Urdwa Dhanurasana (82)
    11. Simhasana (29)
    12. Samakonasana (52)
    13. Suptha Veerasana (24)
    14. Ushtrasana (43)
    15. Bhujangasana (70)
    16. Shalabhasana (74)
    17. Makarasana (78)
    18. Dhanurasana (79)
    19. Marichasana (40)
    20. Hanumanasana (61)
    21. Paryankasana (25)
    22. Shavasana (100)

III. **Pranayama**
    1. Anuloma-Viloma
    2. Ujjayi
    3. Nadishodana

IV. **Meditation**

8. YOGIC EXERCISES FOR BEAUTICIANS AND MODELS

I. **Suryanamaskara:** 13 times with mantras.

II. **Yogasanas**
    1. All standing Yogasana Postures
    2. Simhasana (29)
    3. Ushtrasana (43)
    4. Matsyasana (30)
    5. Lagu Vajrasana (44)
    6. Vrischikasana (94 & 95)
    7. Mayurasana (33)
    8. Sarvangasana (56)
    9. Shirshasana (84)
    10. Paschimothanasana (38)
    11. Bhujangasana (70)
    12. Makarasana (78)
    13. Dhanurasana (all types 79 to 83)
    14. Pincha Mayurasana (92)
    15. Chakrasana (85)
    16. Gandabherundasana (90)

17. Omkarasana (66)
18. Hanumanasana (61)
19. Hanumana Valikilyasana (62)
20. Shavasana (100)

III. Pranayama
All types of Pranayama.

IV. Meditation

V. Herbal/Food Therapy
1. Taking the decoction of Emblic Myrobalans with equal quantity of heart leaved juice (Tinospora cordifolia) mixed together and taken twice daily helps to maintain youthfulness forever.
2. Application of lemon juice to the face and body regularly helps to give fair complexion to the skin.
3. Taking fruit juices, dry fruits provides energy to the body and also helps in beautification of body.
4. Grind arhar dal (cajamus indicus) and make a paste. Apply the paste to the face, hands, legs etc. to improve the complexion of the skin.
5. Apply the juice of cucumber to the face and body to improve the complexion of the body.
6. The application of neem oil extracted from neem leaves helps to increase skin complexion.

9. YOGIC EXERCISES FOR SPORTSMEN/ATHLETES

I. Suryanamaskara: 13 times with mantras.

II. Yogasana
1. All standing Yogasana Postures
2. Sarvangasana (56)
3. Shirshasana (84)
4. Matsyasana (30)
5. Mayurasana (33)
6. Paschimothanasana (38)
7. Angustasana (48)
8. Hanumanasana (61)
9. Samakonasana (52)
10. Shavasana (100)

III. Pranayama
1. Anuloma-Viloma
2. Ujjayi
3. Nadishodhana

IV. Meditation

IMPORTANT YOGIC EXERCISES FOR DAILY PRACTICE
[ONE HOUR EXERCISE]

Yogic Exercises	Breaths	Mins.
I. Suryanamaskara: 13 times with mantras.		10
II. Yogasana		
1. Tadasana (1)	10	½
2. Ardhakatichakrasana (2) (both side)	5+5	½
3. Trikonasana (3) (both side)	6+6	1
4. Uttanasana (13)	9	½
5. Shavasana (100)	12 to 16	1
6. Padmasana (20):		
a) Right leg		
—Parvatasana (32)	10	½
—Simhasana (29)	10	½
b) Left leg—Matsyasana (30)	10	½
7. Shavasana (100)	10	½
8. Viparitha Karni (56)	20	1
9. Sarvangasana (56)	40	½
10. Halasana (57)	10	½
11. Karna Peedasana (97)	10	½
12. Shavasana (100)	20	1
13. Mulabandasana (51)	10	½
14. Janu Shirshasana (36) (both side)	5+5	½
15. Paschimothanasana (38)	10	½
16. Ardha Matsyendrasana (41) (both side) OR Marichasana (40) (Both side)	10+10	1
17. Vajrasana +Ushtrasna (22&43)	5+10	1
18. Suptha Veerasana+Paryankasana (24&25)	5+15	1
19. Pavanamukthasana (96)	2	
20. Bhujangasana (70)	10	½
21. Shalabhasana (74)	5	¼
22. Makarasana (78)	5	¼
23. Dhanurasana (79)	10	½
24. Urdwa Dhanurasana I &II (81&82)	5+5	½
25. Shirshasana (84)	60	2-3
26. Shavasana (100) (Complete relaxation)		15
III. Pranayama		
1. Anuloma-Viloma----------10 rounds		
2. Ujjayi--------------------10 rounds.		
3. Nadishodana-------------9 rounds		
IV. Meditation		5

Note : Here only the important yogic exercises required for daily practice have been mentioned. The yoga practitioner has to perform all the important yogasanas contained in this book. More importantly yoga practitioner has to perform yogic exercises very calmly and with utmost concentration and peace of mind. Then only the good results can be expected.

BIBLIOGRAPHY

1. **Light on Yoga**
   —B. K. S. Iyengar
2. **The Complete Book of Yoga**
   —Sri Anand
3. **Yogic Cure for Common Diseases**
   —Phulgenda Sinha
4. **Yoga Sudha**
   —Journals of Vivekananda Yoga Kendra, Bangalore

Yogasanas and Sadhana

—Dr. Satpal Grover

Explore the Influence of Yoga for Sure Cure!

Yoga is a way of life. It enables us to have multi-dimensional approach to life. Yoga is art as well as science. The practice of yoga can help keeping the body and mind healthy. In fact, in the present day conditions, maintaining good health has become more difficult. Consequently diseases are proliferating.

If you, therefore, wish to keep good health, certain yogic principles have to be observed. If you follow these principles and practice, yoga and yogasanas regularly, it would not be a problem to enjoy full strength & vigour.

Yoga is a great dynamo of power that you have to tap to become a master of yourself and the world. In fact, you have a great power & energy within, provided you can exploit it & make your own to utilize it when required. Yoga is a complete art—it is a science that is capable of giving you physical and mental health. When you have a sound mind and healthy body, you are able to enjoy yourself fully. When you are the master of yourself, you don't have to indulge in any kind of vices.

Keeping that aim in mind Dr. Satpal has written this book, **Yogasanas and Sadhana**, which will surely prove more useful to all the students of yoga. It is hoped that those who practise yoga will derive complete benefit from this revised book and will also extend this benefit to others.

Demy Size • Pages: 104 • Price: Rs. 60/- • Postage: Rs. 15/-

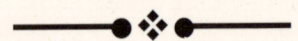

Health Rejuvenating EXERCISES

—Swami Dharmananda Jain

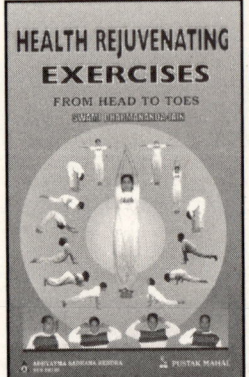

Asanas have an essential role in Preksha meditation. A major objective of meditation is to achieve perfect concentration. Concentration affects and is associated with the digestive system. The practice of asanas leads to an increase in the activity of the digestive system, making them and pranayama indispensable constituents of meditation.

Dharmanandaji is a skilled practitioner of asanas. He has tried to integrate the ancient in contemporary practices. Physiologists are of the opinion that some asanas which put more pressure on a particular organ of the body need not be practised. That is why a few of the old asanas have been set aside and need to be replaced by new ones.

Yogic kriyas have gained wide acceptance because these are easy to perform and involve little effort. The sequence of these exercises has been beautifully arranged in the present booklet, which also clarifies their utility in the context of asanas.

Demy Size • Pages: 52 • Price: Rs. 24/- • Postage: Rs. 10/-

The Joy of Natural Living

—*Luis S.R. Vas & Anita S.R. Vas*

The Joy of Natural Living incorporates research findings on health, psychology, body care and spirituality which emphasise the benefits of natural living. A common theme runs through all the material gathered here. The more you rely on nature and nature therapy in dealing with your physical and mental problems, the more joy you get out of life.

The authors hope the reader will be able to regain natural joy by experimenting with some of the advice from experts presented here which include:

- Coping with stress through relaxation techniques and pleasant and positive thoughts.
- Role of diet in achieving mental & physical well being.
- Safe & successful physical activity program.
- Natural grooming and herbal preparation to attain increased self-confidence.

Demy Size • Pages: 152 • Price: Rs. 80/- • Postage: Rs. 15/-

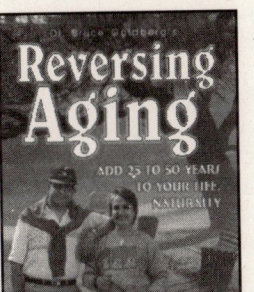

Reversing Aging

—*Dr. Bruce Goldberg*

Aging slowly allows us to enjoy life to the hilt, rather than expend our energies resisting Father Time. The very thought of growing old and the inevitable difficulties usually associated with aging depresses most people. Now science is on the threshold of showing us how aging can be prevented, or at least delayed.

Reversing Aging presents both theory and specific techniques to deal with life's challenges associated with aging. The author, Dr. Bruce Goldberg, has drawn the most accurate and useful information available from the fields of personal grooming, gerontology (the study of aging), nutrition, exercise, biochemistry and alternative medicine to help improve and retain your vigour throughout life.

In the book, you will discover:

- How to use self-hypnosis to slow down the aging process.
- How to take a balanced diet for a longer life.
- How to change your lifestyle to preserve youth.
- How to change aging indicators.
- How to look younger through simple, natural methods.

Demy Size • Pages: 224 • Price: Rs. 80/- • Postage: Rs. 15/-

Meditation

The gateway to enhance your health, mental abilities as well as emotional & spiritual well being

—*Luis S.R. Vas*

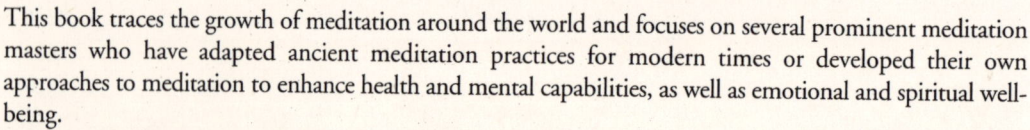

Meditation techniques evolved by Meditation Masters

Meditation is an ancient religious practice, being routinely prescribed in the modern secular society, not just by spiritual masters, but by behavioural scientists, medical practitioners and business consultants. It has found widely varied applications in religious institutions, medical facilities, educational establishments and business organisations. This is a relatively recent development. Less than half a century ago the word meditation, in the sense it is used today, was largely unfamiliar to those outside the Hindu and Buddhist religious traditions.

This book traces the growth of meditation around the world and focuses on several prominent meditation masters who have adapted ancient meditation practices for modern times or developed their own approaches to meditation to enhance health and mental capabilities, as well as emotional and spiritual well-being.

It concludes with a discussion on the benefits of meditation for modern men and women. The reader can try out the various techniques described and decide on the one most suited to his or her own needs.

Demy Size • Pages: 224 • Price: Rs. 88/- • Postage: Rs. 15/-

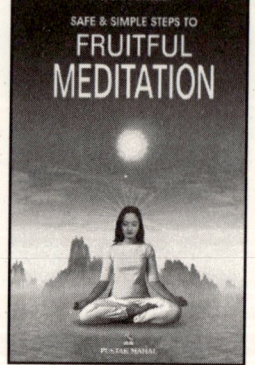

Safe & Simple Steps to Fruitful Meditation

—*By Dr N K Srinivasan*

Meditation is widely accepted as a method to reduce mental tensions and achieve inner peace and tranquillity, leading to spiritual growth. In this book, various techniques are presented in easy step-by-step procedures, starting with simple techniques that can be practised for just a few minutes.

The benefits are clearly described so that the practitioner can track his or her progress. The best traditions of meditation in India are presented so that modern folk with limited background of yoga and Indian philosophy can follow the steps. One can learn these techniques without a personal instructor.

A detailed chapter on *chakras* and *Kundalini yoga* is valuable for serious meditators. The Buddhist meditations, widely used in the West and meant for the awakening inner joy, are described in a separate chapter. Creative visualisation – a meditational technique to achieve practical goals in business life – is described. The book dispels common doubts about the efficacy of meditation and guides and motivates the reader towards the best meditation practices.

Demy Size • Pages: 96 • Price: Rs. 80/- • Postage: Rs. 15/-

YOGA for HEALTH & PERSONALITY

—*Dr. G. Francis Xavier,* PhD

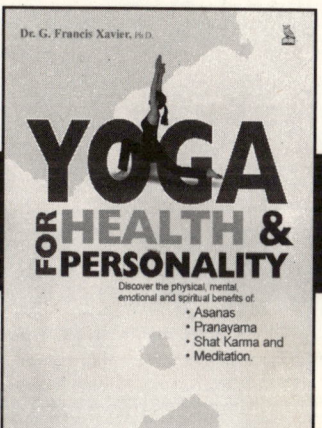

Yoga is a holistic science promoting specific techniques for integrated development of man's entire being—physical, mental, emotional and spiritual. Regular practise of Yoga ensures sound health, sharp intellect, youthful looks, abundant energy, emotional maturity, composure, compassion and spiritual awareness.

This book perhaps the only book that offers all practical aspects of Yoga—Asanas, Pranayama, Shat Karma and meditation. The pages are profusely illustrated with photos of Yogic asanas performed by the author and others, making it easy to follow the step-by-step guidelines explaining the techniques for every posture. The specific benefits of each asana are also stated. Suitable for young and old alike, just half an hour of daily Yoga will help you overcome bad habits, improve your personality and make you a better human being in every aspect.

Big Size • Pages: 124
Price: Rs. 96/- • Postage: Rs. 15/-

82